SIRTFOOD DIET

RECIPES

THE ULTIMATE SIRT DIET COOKBOOK WITH 147 RECIPES TO ACTIVATE YOUR SKINNY GENE, BURN FAT, LOSE WEIGHT AND KEEP IT OFF FOR GOOD

By
LOLA MATTEN

Table of Contents

Introduction

The basic principles of the sirtfood diet were formulated by scientists and nutritionists Aidan Goggins and Glen Matten in 2016. The popularity of the new teaching came in the last year and a half, when it turned out that with the help of the food-diet, Gwyneth Paltrow, Pippa Middleton, and Prince Harry got in shape on the eve of their weddings. In the fall of 2019, it turned out that it was thanks to the food diet that Adele lost as much as 20 kilograms. The publication began to enjoy even greater fame and with it a new diet.

Experts note that the use of vegetables and fruits is encouraged in sirtfood. It is a fairly strict diet with restircted protein content, and in the long run, the latter factor can lead to loss of muscle tissue. Authors of the methodology assure that their diet is, in many ways, one of the aspects of a healthy lifestyle. Sirtfoods are capable of activating proteins in our body, which help us not accumulate fat and fight against free radicals and diseases, and stimulate metabolism, burn fat, and promote loss.

All the plant foods contain bioactive molecules that are good for the body. However, it is good to have a more profound knowledge of the wide variety of Sirtfoods, which includes foods that hardly imagined being part of a weight loss diet. For example, red wine, which contains sugars and alcohol, and chocolate, is a high-calorie and sugary food. Both of them have a bad reputation for healthy eating. In addition to foods such as strawberries, blueberries and citrus fruits, walnuts, buckwheat, red pepper, and green tea, cabbage, radicchio, red onion, and arugula are well suited to a diet. The exceptional peculiarity of this diet, which makes it almost unique, is the fact that it is based on the inclusion and not on the exclusion of food.

They are all foods that are part of the sirtfood diet, born from genetic studies, based on the activation of the "lean gene" to lose weight in a healthy and fast way, preserving energy, muscle tone, and a good mood. Sirtuins are involved in the regulation of metabolism. It deceives the body and sends a signal that makes us believe that we are fasting, that we are entering a period of famine, and that survival is at risk when in reality, it is not, and we are eating.

They transport the fat reserves from the fat cells to the blood to convert them into energy, and they control the inflammatory processes and the cycle of life. This signal from sirtuins activates the genes responsible for survival, all resources are enabled, and all the available energy is used. Free radical damage repaired to protect us from disease, and fat does not accumulate.

The positive effects of foods that activate sirtuins are enough to make a balanced diet. They are foods rich in particular nutrients that help the production of the lean gene faster than our body would normally do. Many Sirtfood diets were launched in the United States to encourage the consumption of foods that activate sirtuins for weight loss, increase energy, reduce stress levels, and extend life expectancy.

Breakfast Recipes

Day 1.   Matcha Green Juice

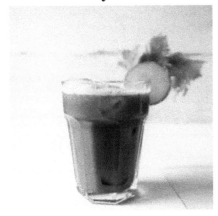

Preparation time: 10 minutes

Cooking time: 0 minutes

Servings: 2

Ingredients:

5 ounces fresh kale

2 ounces fresh arugula

¼ cup fresh parsley

4 celery stalks

1 green apple, cored and chopped

1 (1-inch) piece fresh ginger, peeled

1 lemon, peeled

½ teaspoon matcha green tea

Directions:

Add all ingredients into a juicer and extract the juice according to the manufacturer's method.

Pour into 2 glasses and serve immediately.

Nutrition:

Calories: 113

Fat: 0.6 g

Carbohydrates: 26.71 g

Protein: 3.8 g

Day 2. Celery Juice

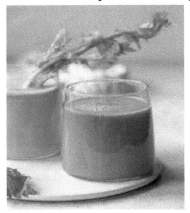

Preparation time: 10 minutes

Cooking time: 0 minutes

Servings: 2

Ingredients:

8 celery stalks with leaves

2 tablespoons fresh ginger, peeled

1 lemon, peeled

½ cup filtered water

Pinch of salt

Directions:

Place all the ingredients in a blender and pulse until well combined.

Through a fine mesh strainer, strain the juice and transfer into 2 glasses.

Serve immediately.

Nutrition:

Calories: 32

Fat: 0.5 g

Carbohydrates: 6.5 g

Protein: 1 g

Day 3.   Kale & Orange Juice

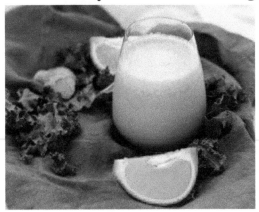

Preparation time: 10 minutes

Cooking time: 0 minutes

Servings: 2

Ingredients:

5 large oranges, peeled and sectioned

2 bunches fresh kale

Directions:

Add all ingredients into a juicer and extract the juice according to the manufacturer's method.

Pour into 2 glasses and serve immediately.

Nutrition:

Calories: 315

Fat: 0.6 g

Carbohydrates: 75.1 g

Protein: 10.3 g

Day 4.   Apple & Cucumber Juice

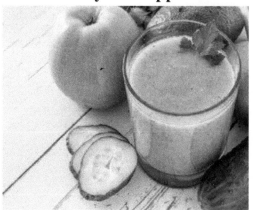

Preparation time: 10 minutes

Cooking time: 0 minutes

Servings: 2

Ingredients:

3 large apples, cored and sliced

2 large cucumbers, sliced

4 celery stalks

1 (1-inch) piece fresh ginger, peeled

1 lemon, peeled

Directions:

Add all ingredients into a juicer and extract the juice according to the manufacturer's method.

Pour into 2 glasses and serve immediately.

Nutrition:

Calories: 230

Fat: 1.1 g

Carbohydrates: 59.5 g

Protein: 3.3 g

Day 5.   Lemony Green Juice

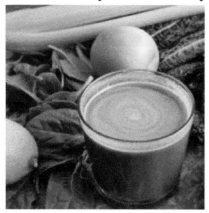

Preparation time: 10 minutes

Cooking time: 0 minutes

Servings: 2

Ingredients:

2 large green apples, cored and sliced

4 cups fresh kale leaves

4 tablespoons fresh parsley leaves

1 tablespoon fresh ginger, peeled

1 lemon, peeled

½ cup filtered water

Pinch of salt

Directions:

Place all the ingredients in a blender and pulse until well combined.

Through a fine mesh strainer, strain the juice and transfer into 2 glasses.

Serve immediately.

Nutrition:

Calories: 196

Fat: 0.6 g

Carbohydrates: 47.9 g

Protein: 5.2 g

Day 6. Kale Scramble

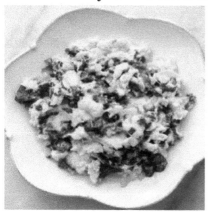

Preparation time: 10 minutes

Cooking time: 6 minutes

Servings: 2

Ingredients:

4 eggs

1/8 teaspoon ground turmeric

Salt and ground black pepper, to taste

1 tablespoon water

2 teaspoons olive oil

1 cup fresh kale, tough ribs removed and chopped

Directions:

In a bowl, add the eggs, turmeric, salt, black pepper, and water and with a whisk, beat until foamy.

In a wok, heat the oil over medium heat.

Add the egg mixture and stir to combine.

Immediately, reduce the heat to medium-low and cook for about 1–2 minutes, stirring frequently.

Stir in the kale and cook for about 3–4 minutes, stirring frequently.

Remove from the heat and serve immediately.

Nutrition:

Calories: 183

Fat: 13.4 g

Carbohydrates: 4.3 g

Protein: 12.1 g

Day 7.   Buckwheat Porridge

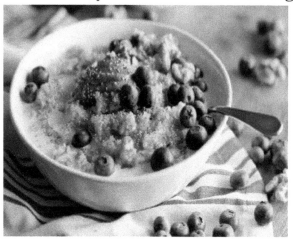

Preparation time: 10 minutes

Cooking time: 15 minutes

Servings: 2

Ingredients:

1 cup buckwheat, rinsed

1 cup unsweetened almond milk

1 cup water

½ teaspoon ground cinnamon

½ teaspoon vanilla extract

1–2 tablespoons raw honey

¼ cup fresh blueberries

Directions:

In a pan, add all the ingredients (except honey and blueberries) over medium-high heat and bring to a boil.

Now, reduce the heat to low and simmer, covered for about 10 minutes.

Stir in the honey and remove from the heat.

Set aside, covered, for about 5 minutes.

With a fork, fluff the mixture, and transfer into serving bowls.

Top with blueberries and serve.

Nutrition:

Calories: 358

Fat: 4.7 g

Carbohydrates: 3.7 g

Protein: 12 g

Day 8.   Blueberry Muffins

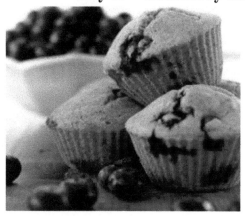

Preparation time: 15 minutes

Cooking time: 20 minutes

Servings: 8

Ingredients

1 cup buckwheat flour

¼ cup arrowroot starch

1½ teaspoons baking powder

¼ teaspoon sea salt

2 eggs

½ cup unsweetened almond milk

2–3 tablespoons maple syrup

2 tablespoons coconut oil, melted

1 cup fresh blueberries

Directions:

Preheat your oven to 350°F and line 8 cups of a muffin tin.

In a bowl, place the buckwheat flour, arrowroot starch, baking powder, and salt, and mix well.

In a separate bowl, place the eggs, almond milk, maple syrup, and coconut oil, and beat until well combined.

Now, place the flour mixture and mix until just combined.

Gently, fold in the blueberries.

Transfer the mixture into prepared muffin cups evenly.

Bake for about 25 minutes or until a toothpick inserted in the center comes out clean.

Remove the muffin tin from oven and place onto a wire rack to cool for about 10 minutes.

Carefully invert the muffins onto the wire rack to cool completely before serving.

Nutrition:

Calories: 136

Fat: 5.3 g

Carbohydrates: 20.7 g

Protein: 3.5 g

Day 9.   Chocolate Waffles

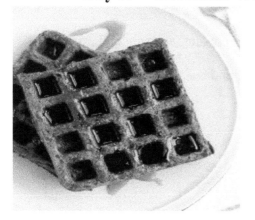

Preparation time: 15 minutes

Cooking time: 24 minutes

Servings: 8

Ingredients

2 cups unsweetened almond milk

1 tablespoon fresh lemon juice

1 cup buckwheat flour

½ cup cacao powder

¼ cup flaxseed meal

1 teaspoon baking soda

1 teaspoon baking powder

¼ teaspoons kosher salt

2 large eggs

½ cup coconut oil, melted

¼ cup dark brown sugar

2 teaspoons vanilla extract

2 ounces unsweetened dark chocolate, chopped roughly

Directions:

In a bowl, add the almond milk and lemon juice and mix well.

Set aside for about 10 minutes.

In a bowl, place buckwheat flour, cacao powder, flaxseed meal, baking soda, baking powder, and salt, and mix well.

In the bowl of almond milk mixture, place the eggs, coconut oil, brown sugar, and vanilla extract, and beat until smooth.

Now, place the flour mixture and beat until smooth.

Gently, fold in the chocolate pieces.

Preheat the waffle iron and then grease it.

Place the desired amount of the mixture into the preheated waffle iron and cook for about 3 minutes, or until golden-brown.

Repeat with the remaining mixture.

Nutrition:

Calories: 295

Fat: 22.1 g

Carbohydrates: 1.5 g

Protein: 6.3 g

Day 10. Moroccan Spiced Eggs

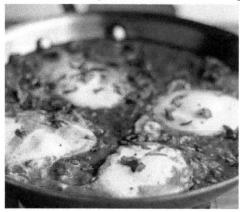

Preparation time: 1 hour

Cooking time: 50 minutes

Servings: 2

Ingredients:

1 tsp. olive oil

1 shallot, stripped and finely hacked

1 red (chime) pepper, deseeded and finely hacked

1 garlic clove, stripped and finely hacked

1 courgette (zucchini), stripped and finely hacked

1 tbsp. tomato purees (glue)

½ tsp. gentle stew powder

¼ tsp. ground cinnamon

¼ tsp. ground cumin

½ tsp. salt

1 × 400g (14oz) can hack tomatoes

1 x 400g (14oz) may chickpeas in water

A little bunch of level leaf parsley (10g (1/3oz)), cleaved

Four medium eggs at room temperature

Directions:

Heat the oil in a pan; include the shallot and red (ringer) pepper and fry delicately for 5 minutes. At that point include the garlic and courgette (zucchini) and cook for one more moment or two. Include the tomato puree (glue), flavour and salt and mix through.

Add the cleaved tomatoes and chickpeas (dousing alcohol and all) and increment the warmth to medium. With the top of the dish, stew the sauce for 30 minutes – ensure it is delicately rising all through and permit it to lessen in volume by around 33%.

Remove from the warmth and mix in the cleaved parsley.

Preheat the grill to 200C/180C fan/350F.

When you are prepared to cook the eggs, bring the tomato sauce up to a delicate stew and move to a little broiler confirmation dish.

Crack the eggs on the dish and lower them delicately into the stew. Spread with thwart and prepare in the grill for 10-15 minutes. Serve the blend in unique dishes with the eggs coasting on the top.

Nutrition:

Calories: 116 kcal

Protein: 6.97 g

Fat: 5.22 g

Carbohydrates: 13.14 g

Day 11. Chilaquiles with Gochujang

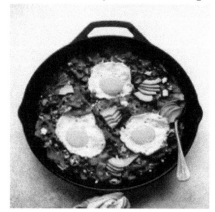

Preparation time: 30 minutes

Cooking time: 20 minutes

Servings: 2

Ingredients:

1 dried ancho Chile

2 cups of water

1 cup squashed tomatoes

2 cloves of garlic

1 teaspoon genuine salt

1/2 tablespoons Gochujang

5 to 6 cups tortilla chips

3 enormous eggs

1 tablespoon olive oil

Directions:

Get the water to heat a pot. I cheated marginally and heated the water in an electric pot and emptied it into the pan.

Add the anchor Chile to the bubbled water and drench for 15 minutes to give it an opportunity to stout up.

When completed, use tongs or a spoon to extricate Chili. Make sure to spare the water for the sauce.

Mix the doused Chili, 1 cup of saved high temp water, squashed tomatoes, garlic, salt and gochujang.

Empty sauce into a large dish and heat 4 to 5 minutes. Heat and include the tortilla chips.

Mix the chips to cover with the sauce. In a different skillet, shower a teaspoon of oil and fry an egg on top, until the whites have settled.

Plate the egg and cook the remainder of the eggs. Sear the eggs while you heat the red sauce.

Top the chips with the seared eggs, cotija, hacked cilantro, jalapeños, onions and avocado. Serve right away.

Nutrition:

Calories: 484 kcal

Protein: 14.55 g

Fat: 18.62 g

Carbohydrates: 64.04 g

Day 12. Twice Baked Breakfast Potatoes

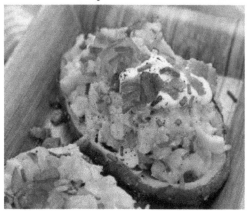

Preparation time: 1 hour 10 minutes

Cooking time: 1 hour

Servings: 2

Ingredients:

2 medium reddish brown potatoes, cleaned and pricked with a fork everywhere

2 tablespoons unsalted spread

3 tablespoons overwhelming cream

4 rashers cooked bacon

4 huge eggs

½ cup destroyed cheddar

Daintily cut chives

Salt and pepper to taste

Directions:

Preheat grill to 400°F.

Spot potatoes straightforwardly on stove rack in the focal point of the grill and prepare for 30 to 45 min.

Evacuate and permit potatoes to cool for around 15 minutes.

Cut every potato down the middle longwise and burrow every half out, scooping the potato substance into a blending bowl.

Gather margarine and cream to the potato and pound into a single unit until smooth — season with salt and pepper and mix.

Spread a portion of the potato blend into the base of each emptied potato skin and sprinkle with one tablespoon cheddar (you may make them remain pounded potato left to snack on).

Add bacon to every half and top with a raw egg.

Spot potatoes onto a heating sheet and come back to the appliance.

Lower broiler temperature to 375°F and heat potatoes until egg whites simply set and yolks are as yet runny.

Top every potato with a sprinkle of the rest of the cheddar, season with salt and pepper and finish with cut chives.

Nutrition:

Calories: 647 kcal

Protein: 30.46 g

Fat: 55.79 g

Carbohydrates: 7.45 g

Day 13. Sirt Muesli

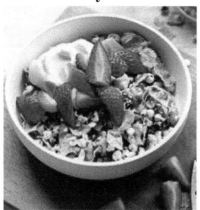

Preparation time: 30 minutes

Cooking time: 0 minutes

Servings: 2

Ingredients:

20g buckwheat drops

10g buckwheat puffs

15g coconut drops or dried up coconut

40g Medjool dates, hollowed and slashed

15g pecans, slashed

10g cocoa nibs

100g strawberries, hulled and slashed

100g plain Greek yoghurt (or vegetarian elective, for example, soya or coconut yoghurt)

Directions:

Blend all the ingredients then put strawberries and yoghurt.

Serve immediately.

Nutrition:

Calories: 334 kcal

Protein: 4.39 g

Fat: 22.58 g

Carbohydrates: 34.35 g

Day 14. Spiced Scramble

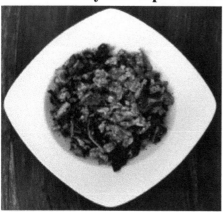

Preparation time: 5 minutes

Cooking time: 5 minutes

Servings: 1

Ingredients:

25g (1oz) kale, finely chopped

2 eggs

1 spring onion (scallion) finely chopped

1 teaspoon turmeric

1 tablespoon olive oil

Sea salt

Freshly ground black pepper

Directions:

Crack the eggs into a bowl. Add the turmeric and whisk them and season with salt and pepper.

Heat the oil in a frying pan, add the kale and spring onions (scallions) and cook until it has wilted.

Pour in the beaten eggs and stir until eggs have scrambled together with the kale.

Nutrition:

Calories: 218

Total Fat: 15.3 g

Cholesterol: 386.9 mg

Sodium: 656.2 mg

Potassium: 243.0 mg

Carbohydrates: 2.8 g

Protein: 17.4 g

Day 15. Cheesy Baked Eggs

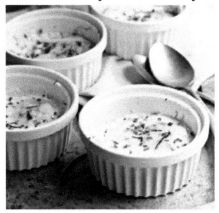

Preparation time: 5 minutes

Cooking time: 15 minutes

Servings: 4

Ingredients:

4 large eggs

75g (3oz) cheese, grated

25g (1oz) fresh rocket (arugula) leaves, finely chopped

1 tablespoon parsley

½ teaspoon ground turmeric

1 tablespoon olive oil

Directions:

Grease each ramekin dish with a little olive oil. Divide the rocket (arugula) between the ramekin dishes then break an egg into each one.

Sprinkle a little parsley and turmeric on top then sprinkle on the cheese.

Place the ramekins in a preheated oven at 220C/425F for 15 minutes, until the eggs are set and the cheese is bubbling.

Nutrition:

Calories: 67

Total Fat: 4 g

Cholesterol: 12 mg

Sodium: 265 mg

Potassium: 84 mg

Total Carbohydrates: 0.2 g

Protein: 8 g

Day 16. Chilled Strawberry and Walnut Porridge

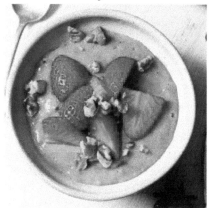

Preparation time: 10 minutes

Cooking time: 12 hours

Servings: 1

Ingredients:

100g (3½ oz) strawberries

50g (2oz) rolled oats

4 walnut halves, chopped

1 teaspoon chia seeds

200mls (7fl oz) unsweetened soya milk

100ml (3½ oz) water

Directions:

Place the strawberries, oats, soya milk and water into a blender and process until smooth.

Stir in the chia seeds and mix well.

Chill in the fridge overnight and serve in the morning with a sprinkling of chopped walnuts. It's simple and delicious.

Nutrition:

Calories: 242

Total Fat: 6 g

Cholesterol: 1.3 mg

Sodium: 37 mg

Potassium: 207 mg

Carbohydrates: 45 g

Protein: 6 g

Day 17. Strawberry & Nut Granola

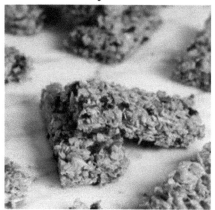

Preparation time: 10 minutes

Cooking time: 50 minutes

Servings: 12

Ingredients:

200g (7oz) oats

250g (9oz) buckwheat flakes

100g (3½ oz) walnuts, chopped

100g (3½ oz) almonds, chopped

100g (3½ oz) dried strawberries

1½ teaspoons ground ginger

1½ teaspoons ground cinnamon

120mls (4fl oz) olive oil

2 tablespoon honey

Directions:

Combine the oats, buckwheat flakes, nuts, ginger and cinnamon.

In a saucepan, warm the oil and honey. Stir until the honey has melted.

Pour the warm oil into the dry ingredients and mix well.

Spread the mixture out on a large baking tray (or two) and bake in the oven at 150C (300F) for around 50 minutes until the granola is golden.

Allow it to cool. Add in the dried berries.

Nutrition:

Calories: 220

Fat: 3 g

Carbohydrates: 44 g

Protein: 6 g

Day 18. Strawberry Buckwheat Pancakes

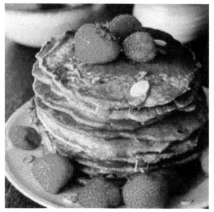

Preparation time: 10 minutes

Cooking time: 20 minutes

Servings: 4

Ingredients:

100g (3½oz) strawberries, chopped

100g (3½ oz) buckwheat flour

1 egg

250mls (8fl oz) milk

1 teaspoon olive oil

1 teaspoon olive oil for frying

Freshly squeezed juice of 1 orange

Directions:

Pour the milk into a bowl and mix in the egg and a teaspoon of olive oil.

Sift in the flour to the liquid mixture until smooth and creamy.

Allow it to rest for 15 minutes. Heat a little oil in a pan and pour in a quarter of the mixture (or to the size you prefer.)

Sprinkle in a quarter of the strawberries into the batter.

Cook for around 2 minutes on each side.

Serve hot with a drizzle of orange juice.

You could try experimenting with other berries such as blueberries and blackberries.

Nutrition:

Calories: 76

Fat: 3 g

Cholesterol: 26 mg

Sodium: 184 mg

Potassium: 17 mg

Carbohydrates: 4 g

Protein: 2 g

Day 19. Poached Eggs & Rocket (Arugula)

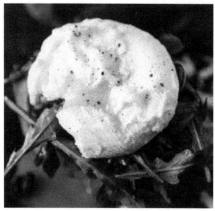

Preparation time: 3 minutes

Cooking time: 5 minutes

Servings: 2

Ingredients:

2 eggs

25g (1oz) fresh rocket (arugula)

1 teaspoon olive oil

Sea salt

Freshly ground black pepper

Directions:

Scatter the rocket (arugula) leaves onto a plate and drizzle the olive oil over them.

Bring a shallow pan of water to the boil, add in the eggs and cook until the whites become firm.

Serve the eggs on top of the rocket and season with salt and pepper.

Nutrition:

Calories: 166

Total Fat: 10 g

Total Carbohydrates: 7 g

Protein: 12 g

Day 20. Chocolate Berry Blend

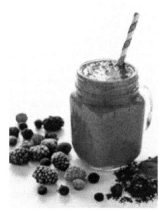

Preparation time: 5 minutes

Cooking time: 5 minutes

Servings: 1

Ingredients:

50g (2oz) blueberries

50g (2oz) strawberries

1 tablespoon 100% cocoa powder or cacao nibs

200mls (7fl oz) unsweetened soya milk

Directions:

Place all of the ingredients into a blender with enough water to cover them and process until smooth.

Nutrition:

Calories: 150

Fat: 9 g

Sodium: 30 mg

Carbohydrates: 17 g

Protein: 3 g

Fiber: 2 g

Sugar: 14 g

Day 21. Mushroom & Red Onion Buckwheat Pancakes

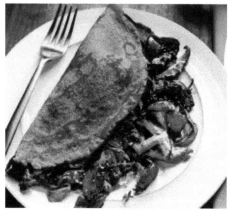

Preparation time: 5 minutes

Cooking time: 10 minutes

Servings: 2

Ingredients:

For the pancakes:

125g (4oz) buckwheat flour

1 egg

150mls (5fl oz) semi-skimmed milk

150mls (5fl oz) water

1 teaspoon olive oil for frying

For the filling:

1 red onion, chopped

75g (3½ oz) mushrooms, sliced

50g (2oz) spinach leaves

1 tablespoon fresh parsley, chopped

1 teaspoon olive oil

50g (2oz) rocket (arugula) leaves

Directions:

Sift the flour into a bowl and mix in an egg.

Pour in the milk and water and mix to a smooth batter. Set aside.

Heat a teaspoon of olive oil in a pan. Add the onion and mushrooms and cook for 5 minutes.

Add the spinach and allow it to wilt. Set aside and keep it warm. Heat a teaspoon of oil in a frying pan and pour in half of the batter.

Cook for 2 minutes on each side until golden.

Spoon the spinach and mushroom mixture onto the pancake and add the parsley.

Fold it over and serve onto a scattering of rocket (arugula) leaves. Repeat for the remaining mixture.

Nutrition:

Calories: 109

Fat: 5 g

Sodium: 61 mg

Potassium: 339 mg

Carbohydrates: 34 g

Protein: 6 g

Day 22. Cream of Broccoli & Kale Soup

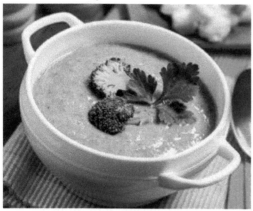

Preparation time: 10 minutes

Cooking time: 30 minutes

Servings: 4

Ingredients:

250g (9oz) broccoli

250g (9oz) kale

1 potato, peeled and chopped

1 red onion, chopped

600mls (1 pint) vegetable stock

300mls (½ pint) milk

1 tablespoon olive oil

Sea salt

Freshly ground black pepper

Directions:

Heat the olive oil in a saucepan, add the onion and cook for 5 minutes.

Add in the potato, kale and broccoli and cook for 5 minutes.

Pour in the stock (broth) and milk and simmer for 20 minutes.

Using a food processor or hand blender, process the soup until smooth and creamy.

Season it with salt and pepper.

Nutrition:

Calories: 123

Total Fat: 7 g

Cholesterol: 16 mg

Sodium: 528 mg

Potassium: 667 mg

Total Carbohydrates: 13.4 g

Protein: 5 g

Day 23. French Onion Soup

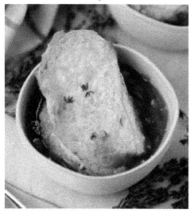

Preparation time: 10 minutes

Cooking time: 55 minutes

Servings: 4

Ingredients:

750g (1¾ lbs) red onions, thinly sliced

50g (2oz) Cheddar cheese, grated (shredded)

12g (½ oz) butter

2 teaspoons flour

2 slices Wholemeal bread

900mls (1½ pints) beef stock (broth)

1 tablespoon olive oil

Directions:

Heat the butter and oil in a large pan. Add the onions and gently cook on a low heat for 25 minutes, stirring occasionally.

Add in the flour and stir well. Pour in the stock (broth) and keep stirring.

Bring to the boil, reduce the heat and simmer for 30 minutes.

Cut the slices of bread into triangles, sprinkle with cheese and place them under a hot grill (broiler) until the cheese has melted.

Serve the soup into bowls and add 2 triangles of cheesy toast on top. Enjoy.

Nutrition:

Calories: 290

Total Fat: 9 g

Total Carbohydrates: 33 g

Protein: 17 g

Day 24. Cheesy Buckwheat Cakes

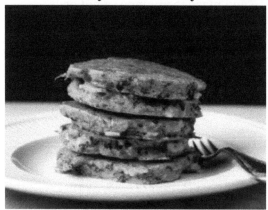

Preparation time: 4 minutes

Cooking time: 4 minutes

Servings: 2

Ingredients:

100g (3½oz) buckwheat, cooked and cooled

1 large egg

25g (1oz) cheddar cheese, grated (shredded)

25g (1oz) Wholemeal breadcrumbs

2 shallots, chopped

2 tablespoons fresh parsley, chopped

1 tablespoon olive oil

Directions:

Crack the egg into a bowl, whisk it then set aside. In a separate bowl combine all the buckwheat, cheese, shallots and parsley and mix well.

Pour in the beaten egg to the buckwheat mixture and stir well.

Shape the mixture into patties. Scatter the breadcrumbs on a plate and roll the patties in them. Heat the olive oil in a large frying pan and gently place the cakes in the oil.

Cook for 3-4 minutes on either side until slightly golden.

Nutrition:

Calories: 240

Total Fat: 4 g

Sodium: 380 mg

Total Carbohydrates: 40 g

Protein: 11 g

Day 25. Lentil Soup

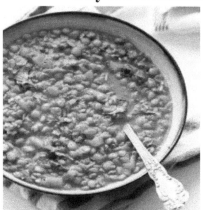

Preparation time: 5 minutes

Cooking time: 55 minutes

Servings: 4

Ingredients:

175g (6oz) red lentils

1 red onion, chopped

1 clove of garlic, chopped

2 sticks of celery, chopped

2 carrots, chopped

½ bird eye chili

1 teaspoon ground cumin

1 teaspoon ground turmeric

1 teaspoon ground coriander (cilantro)

1200mls (2 pints) vegetable stock (broth)

2 tablespoons olive oil

Sea salt

Freshly ground black pepper

Directions:

Heat the oil in a saucepan and add the onion and cook for 5 minutes.

Add in the carrots, lentils, celery, chili, coriander (cilantro), cumin, turmeric and garlic and cook for 5 minutes.

Pour in the stock (broth), bring it to the boil, reduce the heat and simmer for 45 minutes.

Using a hand blender or food processor, puree the soup until smooth.

Season it with salt and pepper. Serve.

Nutrition:

Calories: 194

Total Fat: 1 g

Sodium: 231 mg

Total Carbohydrates: 34 g

Protein: 13

Fiber: 2 g

Day 26. Apple Pancakes

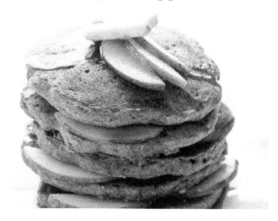

Preparation time: 15 minutes

Cooking time: 24 minutes

Servings: 6

Ingredients:

½ cup buckwheat flour

2 tablespoons coconut sugar

1 teaspoon baking powder

½ teaspoon ground cinnamon

1/3 cup unsweetened almond milk

1 egg, beaten lightly

2 granny smith apples, peeled, cored, and grated

Directions:

In a bowl, place the flour, coconut sugar, and cinnamon, and mix well.

In another bowl, place the almond milk and egg and beat until well combined.

Now, place the flour mixture and mix until well combined.

Fold in the grated apples.

Heat a lightly greased non-stick wok over medium-high heat.

Add desired amount of mixture and with a spoon, spread into an even layer.

Cook for 1–2 minutes on each side.

Repeat with the remaining mixture.

Serve warm with the drizzling of honey.

Nutrition:

Calories 93

Total Fat 2.1 g

Saturated Fat 1 g

Cholesterol 27 mg

Sodium 23 mg

Total Carbohydrates 22 g

Fiber 3 g

Sugar 12.1 g

Protein 2.5 g

Day 27. Matcha Pancakes

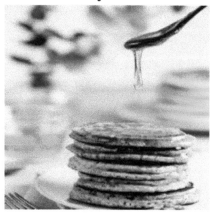

Preparation time: 15 minutes

Cooking time: 24 minutes

Servings: 6

Ingredients:

2 tablespoons flax meal

5 tablespoons warm water

1 cup spelt flour

1 cup buckwheat flour

1 tablespoon matcha powder

1 tablespoon baking powder

Pinch of salt

¾ cup unsweetened almond milk

1 tablespoon olive oil

1 teaspoon vanilla extract

1/3 cup raw honey

Directions:

In a bowl, add the flax meal and warm water and mix well. Set aside for about 5 minutes.

In another bowl, place the flours, matcha powder, baking powder, and salt, and mix well.

In the bowl of flax meal mixture, place the almond milk, oil, and vanilla extract, and beat until well combined.

Now, place the flour mixture and mix until a smooth textured mixture is formed.

Heat a lightly greased non-stick wok over medium-high heat.

Add desired amount of mixture and with a spoon, spread into an even layer.

Cook for about 2–3 minutes.

Carefully, flip the side and cook for about 1 minute.

Repeat with the remaining mixture.

Serve warm with the drizzling of honey.

Nutrition:

Calories 232

Total Fat 4.6 g

Saturated Fat 0.6 g

Cholesterol 0 mg

Sodium 56 mg

Total Carbohydrates 46.3 g

Fiber 5.3 g

Sugar 16.2 g

Protein 6 g

Day 28. Chocolate Muffins

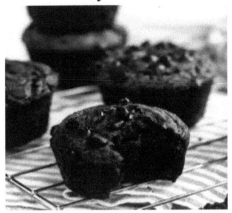

Preparation time: 15 minutes

Cooking time: 20 minutes

Servings: 6

Ingredients:

½ cup buckwheat flour

½ cup almond flour

4 tablespoons arrowroot powder

4 tablespoons cacao powder

1 teaspoon baking powder

½ teaspoon bicarbonate soda

½ cup boiled water

1/3 cup maple syrup

1/3 cup coconut oil, melted

1 tablespoon apple cider vinegar

½ cup unsweetened dark chocolate chips

Directions:

Preheat your oven to 350°F. Line 6 cups of a muffin tin with paper liners.

In a bowl, place the flours, arrowroot powder, baking powder, and bicarbonate of soda, and mix well.

In a separate bowl, place the boiled water, maple syrup, and coconut oil, and beat until well combined.

Now, place the flour mixture and mix until just combined.

Gently, fold in the chocolate chips.

Transfer the mixture into prepared muffin cups evenly.

Bake for about 20 minutes, or until a toothpick inserted in the center comes out clean.

Remove the muffin tin from oven and place onto a wire rack to cool for about 10 minutes.

Carefully invert the muffins onto the wire rack to cool completely before serving.

Nutrition:

Calories 410

Total Fat 28.6 g

Saturated Fat 17.8 g

Sodium 25 mg

Total Carbohydrates 32.5 g

Fiber 5.8 g

Protein 4.6 g

Day 29. Kale & Mushroom Frittata

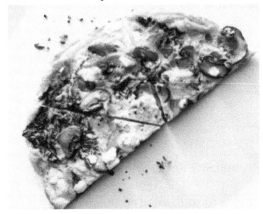

Preparation time: 15 minutes

Cooking time: 30 minutes

Servings: 5

Ingredients:

8 eggs

½ cup unsweetened almond milk

Salt and ground black pepper, to taste

1 tablespoon olive oil

1 onion, chopped

1 garlic clove, minced

1 cup fresh mushrooms, chopped

1½ cups fresh kale, tough ribs removed and chopped

Directions:

Preheat oven to 350ºF.

In a large bowl, place the eggs, coconut milk, salt, and black pepper, and beat well. Set aside.

In a large ovenproof wok, heat the oil over medium heat and sauté the onion and garlic for about 3–4 minutes.

Add the squash, kale, bell pepper, salt, and black pepper, and cook for about 8–10 minutes.

Stir in the mushrooms and cook for about 3–4 minutes.

Add the kale and cook for about 5 minutes.

Place the egg mixture on top evenly and cook for about 4 minutes, without stirring.

Transfer the wok in the oven and bake for about 12–15 minutes or until desired doneness.

Remove from the oven and place the frittata side for about 3–5 minutes before serving.

Cut into desired sized wedges and serve.

Nutrition:

Calories 151

Total Fat 10.2 g

Saturated Fat 2.6 g

Cholesterol 262 mg

Sodium 158 mg

Total Carbohydrates 5.6 g

Fiber 1 g

Sugar 1.7 g

Protein 10.3 g

Day 30. Kale, Apple, and Cranberry Salad

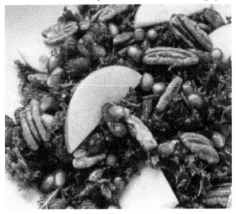

Preparation time: 10 minutes

Cooking time: 15 minutes

Servings: 4

Ingredients:

6 cups fresh baby kale

3 large apples, cored and sliced

¼ cup unsweetened dried cranberries

¼ cup almonds, sliced

2 tablespoons extra-virgin olive oil

1 tablespoon raw honey

Salt and ground black pepper, to taste

Directions:

In a salad bowl, place all the ingredients and toss to coat well.

Serve immediately.

Nutrition:

Calories 253

Total Fat 10.3 g

Saturated Fat 1.2 g

Cholesterol 0 mg

Sodium 84 mg

Total Carbohydrates 40.7 g

Fiber 6.6 g

Sugar 22.7 g

Protein 4.7 g

Lunch Recipes

30.Sticky Chicken Watermelon Noodle Salad

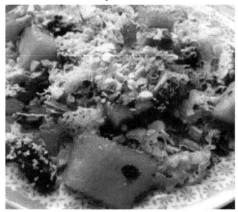

Preparation time: 15 minutes

Cooking time: 20 minutes

Servings: 1

Ingredients:

2 pieces of skinny rice noodles

1/2 tbsp. sesame oil

2 cups Water Melon

Head of bib lettuce

Half of a Lot of scallions

Half of a Lot of fresh cilantro

2 skinless, boneless chicken breasts

1/2 tbsp. Chinese five-spice

1 tbsp. extra virgin olive oil

2 tbsp. sweet skillet

1 tbsp. sesame seeds

A couple of cashews - smashed

Dressing - could be made daily or 2 until

1 tbsp. low-salt soy sauce

1 teaspoon sesame oil

1 tbsp. peanut butter

Half of a refreshing red chili

Half of a couple of chives

Half of a couple of cilantro

Inch limes - juiced

1 small spoonful of garlic

Direction:

In a bowl completely substitute the noodles in boiling drinking water. They are going to soon be carried out in 2 minutes.

On a big sheet of parchment paper, then throw the chicken with pepper, salt, and also the five-spice.

Twist over the newspaper, subsequently celebration and put the chicken using a rolling pin.

Place into the large skillet with 1 tbsp. of olive oil, turning 3 or 4 minutes, until well charred and cooked through.

Drain the noodles and toss with 1 tbsp. of sesame oil onto a sizable serving dish.

Place 50% the noodles into the moderate skillet, stirring frequently until crispy and nice.

Eliminate the Watermelon skin, then slice the flesh to inconsistent balls and then increase the platter.

Reduce the lettuces and cut into small wedges and also half of a whole lot of leafy greens and scatter the dish.

Place another 1 / 2 the cilantro pack, the soy sauce, coriander, chives, peanut butter, and a dab of water, 1 teaspoon of sesame oil, and the lime juice then mix till smooth.

Set the chicken back to heat, garnish with the entire sweet skillet (or my walnut syrup mixture), and toss with the sesame seeds.

Pour the dressing on the salad toss gently with fresh fingers until well coated, then add crispy noodles and then smashed cashews.

Blend chicken pieces and add them to the salad.

Nutrition:

Calories: 694

Total Fat: 33 g

Total Carbohydrates: 22 g

Protein: 14 g

Day 31. Lamb, Butternut Squash and Date Tagine

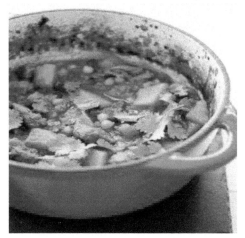

Preparation time: 5 minutes

Cooking time: 1 hour and 15 minutes

Servings: 4

Ingredients:

2 Tsps. coconut oil

1 Red onion, chopped

2cm ginger, grated

3 Garlic cloves, crushed or grated

1 teaspoon chili flakes (or to taste)

2 tsp. cumin seeds

2 teaspoons ground turmeric

1 cinnamon stick

800g lamb neck fillet, cut into 2cm chunks

1/2 tsp. salt

100g Medjool dates, pitted and sliced

400g Tin chopped berries, and half of a can of plain water

500g Butternut squash, chopped into 1cm cubes

400g Tin chickpeas, drained

2 tsp. fresh coriander (and extra for garnish)

Buckwheat, Couscous, flatbread or rice to function

Directions:

Pre heat the oven to 140C.

Drizzle roughly 2 tbsps. coconut oil into a large ovenproof saucepan or cast-iron casserole dish.

Add the chopped onion and cook on a gentle heat, with the lid for around five minutes, until the onions are softened but not too brown.

Insert the grated ginger and garlic, chili, cumin, cinnamon, and garlic. Stir well and cook 1 minute with off the lid. Add a dash of water when it becomes too humid.

Add from the lamb balls. Stir to coat the beef from the spices and onions, and then add the salt chopped meats and berries and roughly half of a can of plain water (100-200ml).

Bring the tagine into the boil and put the lid and put on your skillet for about 1 hour and fifteen minutes.

Add the chopped butternut squash and drained chickpeas. Stir everything together, place the lid back and go back to the oven to the last half an hour of cooking.

When the tagine is able to remove from the oven and then stir fry throughout the chopped coriander.

Nutrition:

Calories: 317

Total Fat: 18 g

Total Carbohydrates: 14 g

Protein: 22 g

Day 32. Turmeric Baked Salmon

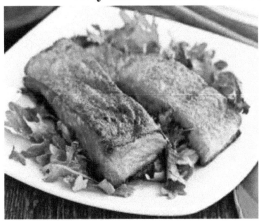

Preparation time: 10 minutes

Cooking time: 10 minutes

Servings: 1

Ingredients:

125-150 g Skinned Salmon

1 tsp. extra virgin coconut oil

1 tsp. Ground turmeric

1/4 Juice of a lemon

1 tsp. extra virgin coconut oil

40 g Red onion, finely chopped

60 g Tinned green peas

1 Garlic clove, finely chopped

1 Cm fresh ginger, finely chopped

1 Bird's eye chili, finely chopped

150 g Celery cut into 2cm lengths

1 tsp. darkened curry powder

130 g Tomato, cut into 8 wedges

100 ml vegetable or pasta stock

1 tbsp. parsley, chopped

Directions:

Heat the oven to 200C / gas mark 6.

Start using the hot celery. Heat a skillet over a moderate --low heat, then add the olive oil then the garlic, onion, ginger, celery, and peppermint.

Fry lightly for 2-3 minutes until softened but not colored, you can add the curry powder and cook for a further minute.

Insert the berries afterward, your lentils and stock, and simmer for 10 seconds. You might choose to increase or reduce the cooking time according to how crunchy you'd like your own sausage.

Meanwhile, mix the garlic olive oil and lemon juice and then rub the salmon.

Set on the baking dish and cook 8 – 10 seconds.

In order to complete, stir the skillet throughout the celery and function with the salmon.

Nutrition:

Calories: 205

Total Fat: 14 g

Cholesterol: 47 mg

Sodium: 622.0 mg

Potassium: 487 mg

Total Carbohydrates: 2 g

Protein: 18 g

Prawn Arrabiata

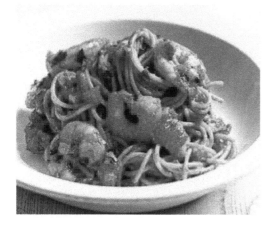

Preparation time: 15 minutes

Cooking time: 35 minutes

Servings:

Ingredients:

125-150 g Beef or cooked prawns (Ideally king prawns)

65 g Buckwheat pasta

1 tablespoon extra-virgin coconut oil

Arrabiata sauce

40 g Red onion, finely chopped

1 Garlic clove, finely chopped

30 g celery, thinly sliced

1 Bird's eye chili, finely chopped

1 tsp. Dried mixed veggies

1 tsp. extra virgin coconut oil

2 Tablespoon White wine (optional)

400 Gram tinned chopped berries

1 tbsp. Chopped parsley

Directions:

Fry the garlic, onion, celery, and peppermint and peppermint blossoms at the oil over moderate-low heat for 1- 2 weeks.

Turn up the heat to medium, bring the wine and cook 1 second.

Add the berries and leave the sauce simmer over moderate-low heat for 20 to half an hour, until it's a great rich texture. In the event you're feeling that the sauce is becoming too thick, simply put in just a very little water.

As the sauce is cooking, attract a bowl of water to the boil and then cook the pasta as per the package directions. Once cooked to your dish, drain, then toss with the olive oil and also maintain at the pan before needed.

If you're utilizing raw prawns, put them into your sauce and cook for a further 3 - 4 minutes, till they've turned opaque and pink, and then add the parsley and function. If you're using cooked prawns, insert them using the skillet, and then bring the sauce to the boil and then function.

Add the cooked pasta into the sauce, then mix thoroughly but lightly and function.

Nutrition:

Calories: 415

Total Fat: 10 g

Total Carbohydrates: 57 g

Protein: 23 g

Day 33. Baked Potatoes with Spicy Chickpea Stew

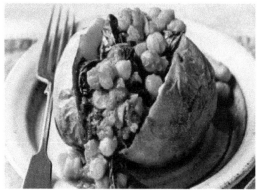

Preparation time: 10 minutes

Cooking time: 1 hour

Servings: 4 - 6

Ingredients:

4 - 6 Celery, pricked all over

2 tsp. coconut oil

2 Red onions, finely chopped

4 Cloves garlic, crushed or grated

2cm ginger, grated

1/2 -2 teaspoons chili flakes (depending on how hot you enjoy stuff)

2 tablespoons cumin seeds

2 tsp. turmeric

Splash Of water

2 x 400g tins chopped tomatoes

2 tablespoons unsweetened cocoa powder (or even cacao)

2 X 400g tins chickpeas including the chick-pea water, do not drain

2 Yellow peppers (or any color you would like), chopped into bite size pieces

2 tablespoons parsley and extra for garnish

Salt And pepper to taste (optional)

Negative Salad (discretionary)

Directions:

Pre heat the oven to 200C, however, you are able to prepare all of your own ingredients.

When the oven is still hot enough to set your lemon potatoes from the oven and cook for 1 hour or so until they do the way you prefer them.

Once the potatoes come from the oven, then place the coconut oil and sliced red onion into a large wide saucepan and cook lightly, with the lid for five minutes until the onions are tender but not brown.

Remove the lid and then add the ginger, garlic, cumin, and simmer. Cook for a further minute on very low heat, then add the garlic and a tiny dab of water and then cook for another moment; just take care never to allow the pan to get too tender.

Add from the berries, cocoa powder (or even cacao), chickpeas (including the chickpea water) and salt.

Allow to the boil, and then simmer on a very low heat for 4-5 seconds before the sauce is thick and unctuous (but do not allow it to burn up). The stew ought to be performed at exactly the exact same period as the legumes.

Finally, Stir at the two tbsp. of parsley, plus a few pepper and salt if you desire, and also serve the stew in addition to the chopped sausage, possibly with a very simple salad.

Nutrition:

Calories: 348

Total Fat: 17 g

Sodium: 148 mg

Potassium: 312 mg

Total Carbohydrates: 41 g

Protein: 7 g

Day 34. Char-grilled Steak

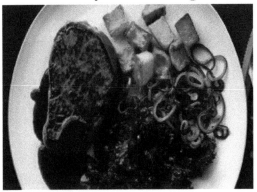

Preparation time:

Cooking time:

Servings:

Ingredients:

5g parsley, finely chopped

100g potatoes, peeled and cut into 2cm dice

50g Lettuce, chopped

1 tbsp. extra virgin coconut oil

50g Red onion, chopped into circles

1 garlic clove, finely chopped

120 - 150g 3.5cm thick beef noodle beef or 2cm-thick sirloin beef

40ml Red wine

150ml Beef inventory

1 tsp. tomato purée

1 tsp. corn flour, dissolved in 1 tablespoon water

Direction:

Heating the oven to 220°C

Put the sausage in a saucepan of boiling water, then return to the boil and then cook 4 minutes, then empty.

Put in a skillet with 1 tbsp. of the oil and then roast in the oven for 4 – 5 minutes. Twist the berries every 10 minutes to ensure even cooking. After cooking, remove from the oven, sprinkle with the chopped parsley, and mix well.

Fry the onion 1 tsp. of the oil over a moderate heat for 5 minutes until tender and well caramelized.

Maintain heat. Steam the kale for 2 - 3 minutes. Stir the garlic lightly in 1/2 tsp. of oil for 1 minute until tender but not colored. Insert the spinach and simmer for a further 1--two minutes, until tender. Maintain heat.

Heat ovenproof skillet until smoking then laid the beef from 1/2 a tsp. of the oil. Then fry from the skillet over a moderate-high temperature in accordance with just how you would like your beef done. If you prefer your beef moderate, it'd be wise to sear the beef and also transfer the pan into a toaster place in 220°C/petrol 7 and then finish the cooking which manner to your prescribed occasions.

Remove the meat from the pan and put aside to break. Add your wine into the skillet to bring any meat up residue. Bubble to decrease the wine by half an hour until syrupy, along with a flavor that is concentrated.

Insert the inventory and tomato purée into the beef pan and bring to the boil, add the corn flour paste to thicken your sauce, then adding it only a little at a time till you've got your preferred consistency.

Stir in just about anyone of those juices out of the dinner that is rested and serve with the roasted lettuce, celery, onion rings, and red berry sauce.

Nutrition:

Calories: 416

Total Fat: 13 g

Total Carbohydrates: 39 g

Protein: 35 g

Day 35. Fruity Curry Chicken Salad

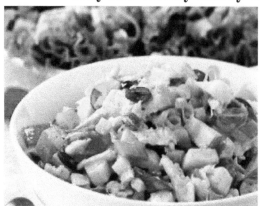

Preparation time: 10 minutes

Cooking time: 10 minutes

Servings: 8

Ingredients

4 skinless, boneless chicken pliers - cooked and diced

1 tsp. celery, diced

4 green onions, sliced

1 golden delicious apple peeled, cored and diced

1/3 cup golden raisins

1/3 cup seedless green grapes, halved

1/2 cup sliced toasted pecans

1/8 tsp. Ground black pepper

1/2 tsp. curry powder

3/4 cup light mayonnaise

Directions:

In a big bowl combine the chicken, onion, celery, apple, celery, celery, pecans, pepper, curry powder, and carrot. Mix altogether.

Nutrition:

Calories: 156

Total Fat: 6 g

Total Carbohydrates: 10 g

Protein: 14 g

Day 36. Zuppa Toscana

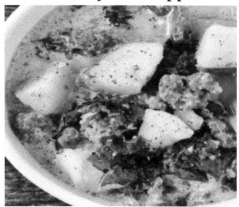

Preparation time: 20 minutes

Cooking time: 1 hour

Servings: 2

Ingredients:

1 lb ground Italian sausage

1 1/4 tsp. crushed red pepper flakes

4 pieces bacon, cut into ½ inch bits

1 big onion, diced

1 tbsp. minced garlic

5 (13.75 oz) can chicken broth

6 celery, thinly chopped

1 cup thick cream

1/4 bunch fresh spinach, tough stems removed

Directions:

Cook that the Italian sausage and red pepper flakes in a pot on medium-high heat until crumbly, browned, with no longer pink, 10 to 15minutes. Drain and put aside.

Cook the bacon at the exact Dutch oven over moderate heat until crispy, about 10 minutes.

Drain leaving a couple of tablespoons of drippings together with all the bacon at the bottom of the toaster. Stir in the garlic and onions cook until onions are tender and translucent, about 5 minutes.

Pour the chicken broth to the pot with the onion and bacon mix; contribute to a boil on high temperature.

Add the berries, and boil until fork-tender, about 20 minutes. Reduce heat to moderate and stir in the cream and also the cooked sausage – heat throughout. Mix the lettuce to the soup before serving.

Nutrition:

Calories: 403

Total Fat: 24 g

Cholesterol: 66 mg

Total Carbohydrates: 32 g

Protein: 15 g

Day 37. Turmeric Chicken & Kale Salad with Honey-Lime Dressing

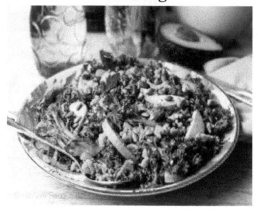

Preparation time: 20 minutes

Cooking time: 10 minutes

Serves: 2

Ingredients:

For the chicken

1 tsp. ghee or 1 tablespoon coconut oil

1/2 moderate brown onion, diced

250 300 grams / 9 oz. Chicken mince or pops upward chicken thighs

1 large garlic clove, finely-chopped

1 tsp. turmeric powder

Optional 1teaspoon lime zest

Juice of 1/2 lime

1/2 tsp. salt

For your salad:

6 broccoli 2 or two cups of broccoli florets

2 tbsp. pumpkin seeds (pepitas)

3 big kale leaves, stalks removed and sliced

Optional 1/2 avocado, chopped

Bunch of coriander leaves, chopped

Couple of fresh parsley leaves, chopped

For your dressing:

3 tbsp. lime juice

1 small garlic clove, finely diced or grated

3 tbsp. extra virgin coconut oil

1 tsp. raw honey

1/2 tsp. whole grain or Dijon mustard

1/2 tsp. sea salt

Directions:

Heat the ghee or coconut oil at a tiny skillet pan above medium-high heat. Bring the onion and then sauté on moderate heat for 45 minutes, until golden.

Insert the chicken blossom and garlic and simmer for 2-3 minutes on medium-high heat, breaking it all out.

Add the garlic, lime zest, lime juice, and salt and soda and cook stirring often, to get a further 3-4 minutes. Place the cooked mince aside.

As the chicken is cooking, add a little spoonful of water. Insert the broccoli and cook 2 minutes. Rinse under warm water and then cut into 3-4 pieces each.

Insert the pumpkin seeds into the skillet out of the toast and chicken over moderate heat for two minutes, stirring often to avoid burning and season with a little salt. Set aside. Raw pumpkin seeds will also be nice to utilize.

Put chopped spinach at a salad bowl and then pour over the dressing table. With the hands, massage and toss the carrot with the dressing table. This will dampen the lettuce, a lot similar to what citrus juice will not steak or fish Carpaccio– it "hamburgers" it marginally.

Finally, toss throughout the cooked chicken, broccoli, fresh herbs, pumpkin seeds, and avocado pieces.

Nutrition:

Calories: 418

Total Fat: 21 g

Total Carbohydrates: 10 g

Protein: 46 g

Day 38. Buckwheat Noodles with Chicken Kale & Miso Dressing

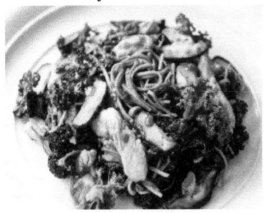

Preparation time: 15 minutes

Cooking time: 15 minutes

Serves: 2

Ingredients:

For the noodles:

2 3 handfuls of kale leaves (removed from the stem and fully trimmed)

150 g / 5 oz buckwheat noodles (100 percent buckwheat, no wheat)

34 shiitake mushrooms, chopped

1 tsp. coconut oil or ghee

1 brown onion, finely diced

1 moderate free-range chicken, chopped or diced

1 red chili, thinly chopped (seeds out based on how hot you want it)

2 large garlic cloves, finely-chopped

23 tbsp. tamari sauce (fermented soy sauce)

For your miso dressing:

1 ½ tbsp. fresh organic miso

1 tbsp. tamari sauce

1 tbsp. peppermint oil

1 tbsp. lime or lemon juice

1 tsp. sesame oil (optional)

Directions:

Bring a medium saucepan of water. Insert the kale and cook 1 minute, until slightly wilted.

Remove and put aside but keep the water and put it back to boil. Insert the soba noodles and cook according to the package directions (usually about five minutes).

Rinse under warm water and place aside. Pan press the shiitake mushrooms at just a very little ghee or coconut oil (about a tsp.) for 23 minutes, until lightly browned on each side. Sprinkle with sea salt and then place aside.

In the exact skillet, warm olive oil ghee over medium-high heating system. Sauté onion and simmer for 2 3 minutes and add the chicken bits.

Cook five minutes over medium heat; stirring a few days, you can put in the garlic, tamari sauce and just a tiny dab of water. Cook for a further 2-3 minutes, stirring often until chicken is cooked through.

Add the carrot and soba noodles and chuck throughout the chicken to heat up.

Mix the miso dressing and scatter on the noodles before eating; in this manner, you can retain dozens of enzymes that are beneficial at the miso.

Nutrition:

Calories: 190

Total Fat: 0.5 g

Sodium: 420 mg

Total Carbohydrates: 38 mg

Protein: 8 g

Day 39. Kale and Red Onion Dhal with Buckwheat

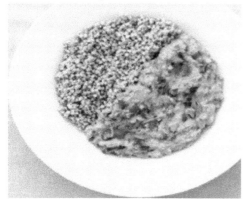

Preparation time: 5 minutes

Cooking time: 25 minutes

Servings: 4

Ingredients:

1 tbsp. coconut oil

1 small red onion, chopped

3 garlic cloves, crushed or grated

2 cm lemon, grated

1birds eye chili deseeded and finely chopped

2 tsp. turmeric

2 teaspoons garam masala

160g red lentils

400ml coconut milk

200ml water

100g kale (or lettuce is a terrific alternative)

160g buckwheat (or brown rice)

Directions:

Put the coconut oil in a large, deep saucepan and then add the chopped onion. Cook on very low heat, with the lid for five minutes until softened.

Insert the ginger, garlic, and chili and cook 1 minute.

Insert the garlic, garam masala and a dash of water and then cook for 1 minute.

Insert the reddish peas, coconut milk, and also 200ml water (try so only by half filling the coconut milk could with water and stirring it in the saucepan).

Mix everything together thoroughly and then cook for 20 minutes over a lightly heat with the lid. Stir occasionally and add just a little bit more water in case the dhal starts to stick.

After 20 seconds, add the carrot, stir thoroughly and then replace the lid, then cook for a further five minutes (1-2 minutes if you are using spinach)

Around 1-5 minutes ahead of the curry is ready, set the buckwheat at a medium saucepan and then put in lots of warm water. Bring back the water to the boil and then cook for 10 minutes (or only a little longer in case you would rather your buckwheat softer. Drain the buckwheat using a sieve and serve with the dhal.

Nutrition:

Calories: 151

Total Fat: 3 g

Sodium: 51.7 mg

Potassium: 531 mg

Total Carbohydrates: 23 g

Protein: 10 g

Day 40. Farinata with Zucchini and Shallot

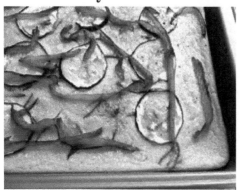

Preparation time: 15 minutes

Cooking time: 40 minutes

Servings: 4

Ingredients:

400 ml of water

125 g of chickpea flour

60 g of Evo oil

8 g of salt

1 zucchini

1 shallot

Directions:

Put the water in a container; gradually add the flour mixing with the whisk to avoid creating lumps.

Add the oil, salt, chopped shallot, zucchini cut into rounds and keep stirring until the mixture is well blended.

Pour it all into a round baking tray greased with a drizzle of oil. Cook at 250° for 30-40 minutes.

Once it's out of the oven, let it cool before you serve it.

Nutrition:

Calories: 129

Total Fat: 6 g

Sodium: 250 mg

Potassium: 195 mg

Total Carbohydrates: 13 g

Protein: 5 g

Day 41. Stuffed with Vegetables

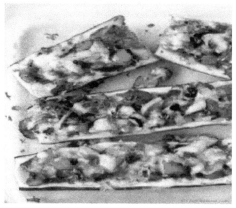

Preparation time: 5 minutes

Cooking time: 15 minutes

Servings: 2

Ingredients:

4 large spoons of chickpea flour

2 level teaspoons of powdered vegetable broth preparation

Sunflower seed oil

300 g mixed vegetables already cooked (e.g. a ratatouille or any other vegetable mix)

Directions:

Mix with a whisk the chickpea flour and the powdered cube, adding water to obtain a rather liquid but still creamy consistency.

Swirl the vegetables with a little sunflower oil and, once heated, pour the batter. For a crispier omelet, the batter layer must be only a few mm thick (maximum one cm, when the filling is abundant).

Cook over low heat on one side until the top has thickened as well. At this point turn with the method you prefer and complete the cooking on the other side.

Nutrition:

Calories: 171

Total Fat: 5 g

Sodium: 225 mg

Potassium: 390 mg

Total Carbohydrates: 25 g

Protein: 5 g

Day 42. Zucchini Dumplings

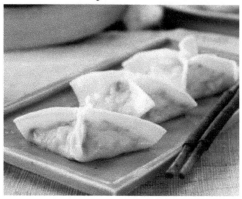

Preparation time: 15 minutes

Cooking time: 1 hour

Servings: 4

Ingredients:

2 zucchini

1 vegan puff pastry for savory pies

8 pitted green olives

Sunflower seeds

1 onion

Pepper

Oil

Directions:

Cut the zucchini into thin slices, put them in the non-stick pan with a drizzle of oil (very little) and simmer them with the lid for about 30 minutes, until well cooked.

Roll out the puff pastry and divide it into 4 parts. Chop the olives; add the chopped onion and some sunflower seeds.

In a small cup place some zucchini (just enough for a dumpling) and add a quarter of the chopped olives, mix and place on the puff pastry.

Add pepper and a drizzle of oil. Repeat the operation for the 4 dumplings, then close them by joining the corners and bake for 30 minutes.

You can also use other vegetables instead of zucchini.

Nutrition:

Calories: 240

Total Fat: 8 g

Total Carbohydrates: 26 g

Protein: 10 g

Day 43. Sponge Beans with Onion

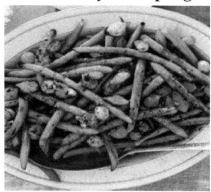

Preparation time: 5 minutes

Cooking time: 1 hour and 30 minutes

Servings: 2

Ingredients:

250 g boiled Spanish beans

1 red onion

1 tablespoon parsley

Salt

2 tablespoons of oil

1 teaspoon of apple vinegar

1 teaspoon of dried oregano or 5 fresh oregano leaves

Directions:

Cut the onion into thin slices and cook it for a minute with a tablespoon of water in the microwave at full power.

Combine all the ingredients in a bowl and leave to rest a couple of hours before serving, stirring a couple of times so that the beans take on the flavour of the seasoning.

Nutrition:

Calories: 250

Total Fat: 7 g

Total Carbohydrates: 36 g

Protein: 5 g

Day 44.   Cannellini Beans

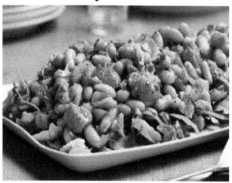

Preparation time: 5 minutes

Cooking time: 25 minutes

Servings: 1

Ingredients:

2 cloves of garlic, minced

2 sage leaves

2 tablespoons of extra virgin olive oil

Boiled cannellini beans

Fresh well ripe tomatoes

Salt and pepper

Directions:

Cook for 2-3 minutes in a pan with oil, garlic and sage.

Then add the tomatoes, cut into segments, and let them brown for a couple of minutes.

Add the beans, salt and pepper to taste, stir.

Cook in a covered pot for 20 minutes, checking and turning occasionally. Serve hot.

Nutrition:

Calories: 320

Total Fat: 7 g

Total Carbohydrates: 54 g

Protein: 18 g

Day 45. Diced Tofu and Lentils

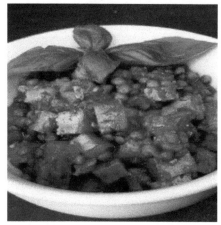

Preparation time: 5 minutes

Cooking time: 30 minutes

Servings: 2

Ingredients:

200 g of tofu cake

Soy sauce (shoyu)

Extra virgin olive oil

Onion

Sprig of rosemary

2 tablespoons of chopped chili pepper

50 g of red lentils

Vegetable stock

Breadcrumbs

Directions:

Marinate the diced tofu for half an hour in the soy sauce, adding a little water to cover it.

In the meantime, boil the red lentils, washed in the vegetable stock for about 20 minutes, until they are soft enough and the stock has dried a bit.

Sauté 2 tablespoons of chili pepper then diced onion and rosemary in olive oil until the onion is golden brown.

Add the tofu with some of the marinating shoyu and after a few minutes also the lentils with very little broth.

Let everything shrink with the lid and over low heat and to thicken add 2 tablespoons of breadcrumbs.

Nutrition:

Calories: 63

Total Fat: 3 g

Total Carbohydrates: 2 g

Fiber: 1 g

Protein: 8 g

Day 46. Seitan and Lentils

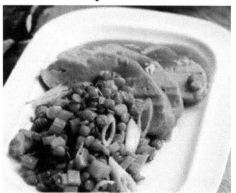

Preparation time: 5 minutes

Cooking time: 10 minutes

Servings: 2

Ingredients:

4 slices of seitan

1 box of lentils

Half onion

1 tablespoon of soy cream

Salt and pepper

1 tablespoon of extra virgin olive oil

Handful of fresh parsley

Turmeric (optional)

Directions:

Chop the onion and cook it in oil. Cut the seitan into cubes.

When it is well coloured - but not burnt - add the seitan cubes and, after a few minutes, add the lentils drained and well washed.

Add salt and pepper and sauté with a little hot water.

Finish with the cream, turmeric and chopped parsley, cook for a few more minutes and then serve with a nice fresh salad and toasted whole meal bread.

Nutrition:

Calories: 120

Total Fat: 6 g

Total Carbohydrates: 15 g

Protein: 60 g

Day 47. Zucchini Croquettes

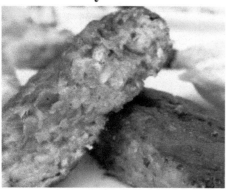

Preparation time: 5 minutes

Cooking time: 20 minutes

Servings: 3

Ingredients:

500 g zucchini

2 slices of bread box

2 tablespoons of yeast

2 tablespoons of breadcrumbs

4 tablespoons of oat flakes

1/2 glass of soya milk

Nutmeg

Directions:

Wash the zucchini, trim them and scratch them with the vegetable grater; dip the slices of bread in soy milk, heat over very low heat, squeeze them and add them to the zucchini.

Add the baking powder, breadcrumbs, oatmeal flakes, nutmeg and salt.

Mix well, form croquettes with wet hands, compact them well and fry in hot oil.

Drain and serve hot. Raw zucchini tend to purge water, so if the mixture is too moist increase the quantity of oat flakes, otherwise these very delicate croquettes could flake during cooking.

Nutrition:

Calories: 228

Total Fat: 20 g

Total Carbohydrates: 11 g

Protein: 16 g

Day 48. Leeks and Mushrooms Crepes

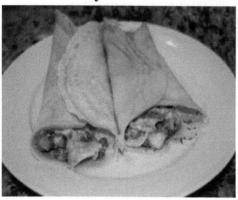

Preparation time: 5 minutes

Cooking time: 25 minutes

Servings: 2

Ingredients:

80 g white flour

20 g of chickpea flour

200 ml of soy milk

100 g of sliced and cooked champignons mushrooms

2 leeks (including the pale green part)

Soya cream

Chives

Garlic powder

Directions:

Mix the two flours in a bowl, and then add the milk a little at a time, stirring with a whisk to avoid the formation of lumps. At pleasure, salt the dough.

Fry the thinly sliced leeks in a frying pan. When they are tender, add the mushrooms and stir for a few minutes.

Add a little soy cream, let it set aside. In the meantime, prepare the crepes: oil a non-stick pan for crepes with the special brush and pour half the mixture, taking care to cover the entire surface of the pan in a thin layer.

Let the other side cozy up, turn and cook too. Stuff it with half the stuffing and roll it up.

Repeat the operation for the second crêpe. In a small bowl, mix soy cream with salt, pepper, chives and garlic powder.

Pour the sauce over the pancakes when serving.

Nutrition:

Calories: 160

Total Fat: 4 g

Sugar: 3 g

Total Carbohydrates: 27 g

Protein: 4 g

Day 49. Herb Crepes

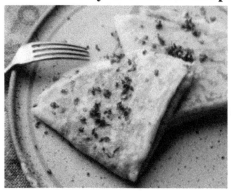

Preparation time: 5 minutes

Cooking time: 25 minutes

Servings: 2

Ingredients:

1/2 cup of flour

1/2 a cup of whole meal flour

3/4 glass of rice milk

Spices to taste

Bunch of chives

Pinch of salt

Pinch of pepper

1 tablespoon of oil

Directions:

Mix all the ingredients in a bowl, starting with the solid ones, including chopped chives.

Gradually add the rice milk until it reaches the right consistency (not too liquid or too thick; if necessary, stretch with a little water).

Grease the pan with the oil you prefer or with a diced vegetable butter, pour one ladle of dough at a time, which will be cooked on both sides until it is golden brown.

You can add a filling as you like or enjoy them naturally.

Nutrition:

Calories: 150

Total Fat: 5 g

Total Carbohydrates: 25 g

Protein: 5 g

Day 50. Baked Cauliflower

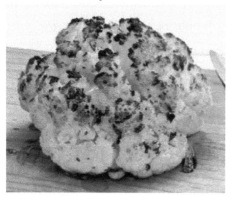

Preparation time: 5 minutes

Cooking time: 20 minutes

Servings: 4

Ingredients:

Cauliflower

Red pepper

Vegan béchamel or soy cream

Handful of breadcrumbs

Fresh chopped parsley

Halls

Herbs (optional)

Directions:

Clean, wash and boil a cauliflower in salted water (a handful of salt). In the meantime, wash and roast a red pepper and, once ready and cooled, remove the skin, open it, clean it from the seeds, reduce it to rags and salt it.

Proceed with the preparation of the vegan béchamel or, alternatively, use soya cream.

Mix the cream and peppers and heat over low heat for 2 minutes, until the mixture is mixed. At discretion, combine herbs.

Place the cauliflower in an earthenware bowl, pour over the cream with the peppers and proceed with a sprinkling of breadcrumbs and chopped fresh parsley. Put in the oven until golden brown.

Nutrition:

Calories: 107

Total Fat: 9 g

Sodium: 740 mg

Potassium: 180 mg

Total Carbohydrates: 6 g

Protein: 3 g

Day 51. Tofu Sticks

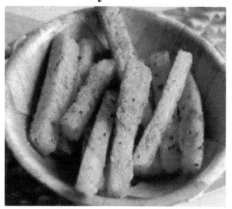

Preparation time: 5 minutes

Cooking time: 15 minutes

Servings: 2

Ingredients:

A brick of tofu

2 tablespoons of chickpea flour

2 tablespoons of corn flour

1 tablespoon of baking powder in flakes

Salt, oregano, paprika oil to fry

1/2 lemon

Directions:

Cut the tofu cake in order to obtain the 'sticks', that is slices 5cm long and about 1 cm thick.

Prepare in a bowl a batter of water and chickpea flour thick enough.

In another bowl mix corn flour and yeast flakes, adding a little salt, oregano, paprika (or other spices to taste).

Pass the slices of tofu one by one in the chickpea batter and then in the corn flour with yeast flakes pressing well with your fingers to cover well.

Heat the oil in a pan and brown them on both sides. After placing them on absorbent paper, spray with drops of lemon juice.

Nutrition:

Calories: 84

Total Fat: 4 g

Sodium: 25 mg

Potassium: 79 mg

Total Carbohydrates: 5 g

Protein: 7 g

Day 52. Pizzaiola Steak

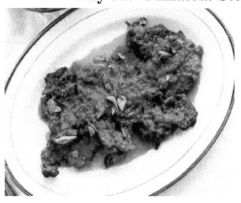

Preparation time: 10 minutes

Cooking time: 50 minutes

Servings: 2

Ingredients:

10 dehydrated soya steaks

1 onion

400 ml of tomato puree

Evo oil

Halls

1 pinch of whole cane sugar

Oregano

Directions:

Soak the soya steaks for 20-30 minutes (as they will float, after 10-15 minutes, turn them on the other side).

Drain them well, pour them in a non-stick pan with some evo oil and chopped onion; brown them for a few minutes.

Pour in the tomato puree, salt, sugar, a drop of water and cook it all covered for 15-20 minutes, stirring occasionally. If the tomato becomes too dry during cooking, add more water. When cooked, add some oregano.

Nutrition:

Calories: 318

Total Fat: 13 g

Cholesterol: 50 mg

Sodium: 600 mg

Total Carbohydrates: 15 g

Protein: 30 g

Day 53. Chicken and Kale with Spicy Salsa

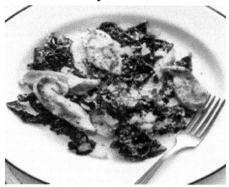

Preparation time: 10 minutes

Cooking time: 50 minutes

Servings: 1

Ingredients:

1 skinless, boneless chicken filet/breast

¼ cup buckwheat

1⁄4 lemon, juiced

1 tbsp. extra virgin olive oil

1 cup kale, chopped

1/2 red onion, sliced

1 tsp. fresh ginger, chopped

2 tsp. ground turmeric

Salsa:

1 tomato

3 sprigs of parsley, chopped

1 tbsp. chopped capers

1 chili, deseeded and minced use less if desired

Juice of 1⁄4 lemon

Directions:

Chop all ingredients above, just for the salsa, and set aside in a bowl.

Pre-eat the oven to 425 F.

Add a teaspoon of the turmeric, the lemon juice and a little oil to the chicken, cover and set aside for 10 minutes.

In a hot pan, slide the chicken and marinade. Cook for 2-3 minutes each side, on high to sear it.

Slide it all onto a baking-safe dish and for cook for about 20 minutes or until cooked.

Lightly steam the kale in a steamer, or on the stovetop with a lid and some water, for about 5 minutes. You want to wilt the kale, not boil or burn it.

Sautee the red onions and ginger, and after 4-5 minutes, add the cooked kale and stir for 1 minute.

Cook the buckwheat, adding in the turmeric. Serve the chicken along with the buckwheat, kale, and spicy salsa.

Nutrition:

Calories: 300

Total Fat: 11 g

Total Carbohydrates: 10 g

Protein: 35 g

Day 54. Shiitake Stew

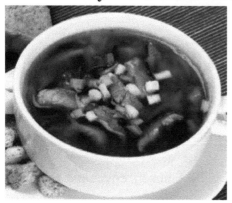

Preparation time: 10 minutes

Cooking time: 3 – 4 hours

Servings: 8

Ingredients:

3 garlic cloves, minced

2 cups chopped onions

1/2 cup olive oil

Salt & 1 tsp. ground pepper to taste

4 cups vegetable broth

2 pounds dry shiitake mushrooms

Directions:

Put ingredients in the slow cooker. Cover and cook on low for 3 to 4 hours.

Nutrition:

Calories: 140

Total Fat: 3 g

Total Carbohydrates: 30 g

Protein: 5 g

Day 55. Chili Con Carne

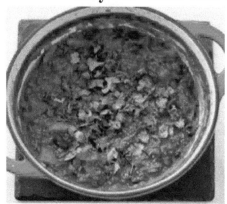

Preparation time: 5 minutes

Cooking Time: 45 minutes

Servings: 4

Ingredients:

1 red onion, chopped

3 cloves of garlic, finely chopped

2 Tai chilies, finely chopped

1 tablespoon of olive oil

1 tablespoon turmeric

1 tablespoon cumin

400g minced beef

150ml red wine

1 red pepper, seeded and diced

2 cans of small tomatoes (400ml each)

1 tablespoon of tomato paste

1 tablespoon cocoa powder without sugar

150g canned kidney beans, drained

300ml beef broth

5g coriander green, chopped

5g parsley, chopped

160g buckwheat

Directions:

Sauté the onions, garlic and chilies in olive oil in a high frying pan or in a frying pan at medium heat. After three minutes add cumin and turmeric and stir.

Then add the minced meat and fry until everything is brown. Add the red wine, bring to the boil and reduce by half.

Add the peppers, tomatoes, tomato paste, cocoa, kidney beans and stock, stir and cook for an hour. Add a little water or broth if the chili is too dry.

Cook buckwheat according to the Directions on the packet and serve sprinkled with the chilies and fresh herbs.

Nutrition:

Calories: 101

Total Fat: 3 g

Cholesterol: 50 mg

Total Carbohydrates: 10 g

Protein: 11 g

Day 56. Mussels in Red Wine Sauce

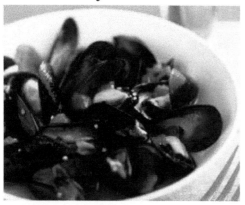

Preparation time: 5 minutes

Cooking Time: 50 minutes

Servings: 2

Ingredients:

800g 2lb mussels

2 x 400g 14 oz tins of chopped tomatoes

25g 1oz butter

1 tablespoon fresh chives, chopped

1 tablespoon fresh parsley, chopped

1 bird's-eye chili, finely chopped

4 cloves of garlic, crushed

400 ml 14fl. oz red wine

Juice of 1 lemon

364 calories per serving

Directions:

Wash the mussels, remove their beards and set them aside. Heat the butter in a large saucepan and add in the red wine.

Reduce the heat and add the parsley, chives, chili and garlic whilst stirring. Add in the tomatoes, lemon juice and mussels.

Cover the saucepan and cook for 2-3 minutes. Remove the saucepan from the heat and take out any mussels which haven't opened and discard them. Serve and eat immediately.

Nutrition:

Calories: 380

Total Fat: 15 g

Cholesterol: 95 mg

Total Carbohydrates: 17 g

Protein: 35 g

Day 57. Roast Balsamic Vegetables

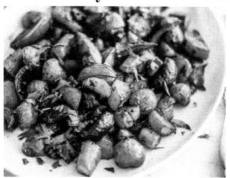

Preparation time: 5 minutes

Cooking time: 45 minutes

Servings: 2

Ingredients:

4 tomatoes, chopped

2 red onions, chopped

3 sweet potatoes, peeled and chopped

100g 3½ oz red chicory or if unavailable, use yellow

100g 3½ oz kale, finely chopped

300g 11oz potatoes, peeled and chopped

5 stalks of celery, chopped

1 bird's-eye chili, de-seeded and finely chopped

2 tablespoons fresh parsley, chopped

2 tablespoons fresh coriander cilantro chopped

3 tablespoons olive oil

2 tablespoons balsamic vinegar 1 teaspoon mustard

Sea salt

Freshly ground black pepper

310 calories per serving

Directions:

Place the olive oil, balsamic, mustard, parsley and coriander cilantro into a bowl and mix well.

Toss all the remaining ingredients into the dressing and season with salt and pepper.

Transfer the vegetables to an ovenproof dish and cook in the oven at 200C/400F for 45 minutes.

Nutrition:

Calories: 123

Total Fat: 3 g

Sodium: 45 mg

Total Carbohydrates: 24 g

Protein: 5 g

Day 58. Honey Chili Squash

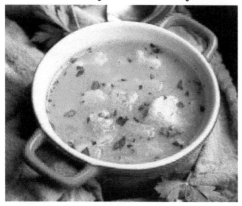

Preparation time: 5 minutes

Cooking time: 20 minutes

Servings: 2

Ingredients:

2 red onions, roughly chopped 2.5cm

1 inch chunk of ginger root, finely chopped

2 cloves of garlic

2 bird's-eye chilies, finely chopped

1 butternut squash, peeled and chopped

100 ml 3½ fl. oz vegetable stock broth

1 tablespoon olive oil

Juice of 1 orange

Juice of 1 lime

2 teaspoons honey

Directions:

Warm the oil into a pan and add in the red onions, squash chunks, chilies, garlic, ginger and honey. Cook for 3 minutes.

Squeeze in the lime and orange juice. Pour in the stock broth, orange and lime juice and cook for 15 minutes until tender.

Nutrition:

Calories: 214

Total Fat: 6 g

Cholesterol: 60 mg

Total Carbohydrates: 24 g

Protein: 18 g

Dinner Recipes

59.Bang-Bang Chicken Noodle Stir-fry

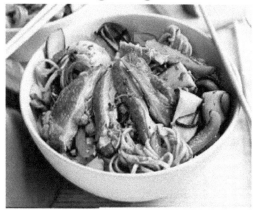

Preparation time: 20 minutes

Cooking time: 1 hour and 10 minutes

Servings: 4

Ingredients:

1 tablespoon sunflower oil

750g package chicken thighs, boned, any surplus skin trimmed

250g frozen chopped mixed peppers

Inch courgette, peeled into ribbons, seeded center chopped

1 chicken stock cube

250g pack moderate egg yolks

4 garlic cloves, finely chopped

1/2 tsp. crushed chilies, and additional to serve (optional)

4 tablespoons reduced-salt soy sauce

2 tsp. caster sugar

1 lime, zested, 1/2 juiced, 1/2 slice into wedges to function

Directions:

Heat the oil in a skillet on medium-low warmth. Fry the chicken skin-side down to 10 minutes or until your skin is emptied.

Flip and simmer for 10 minutes, or until cooked. Transfer to a plate cover loosely with foil.

Reheat the wok over a high temperature, add the peppers and sliced courgette; simmer for 5 minutes.

Meanwhile, bring a bowl of water to the boil, and then crumble in the stock block, adding the noodles. Simmer for 45 minutes until cooked, and then drain well.

Insert the garlic and crushed chilies into the wok; simmer for 2 minutes. In a bowl, mix the soy sugar and the lime juice and zest.

Enhance the wok, bubble 2 minutes; you can add the courgette noodles and ribbons. Toss with tongs to coat in the sauce.

Cut the chicken into pieces. Divide the noodles between 4 bowls and top with the chicken. Serve with the lime wedges along with extra crushed chilies, in case you prefer.

Nutrition:

Calories: 710

Total Fat: 30 g

Total Carbohydrates: 7 g

Protein: 40 g

Day 59. Pesto Salmon Pasta Noodles

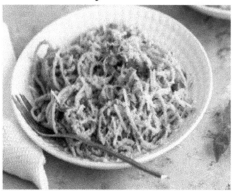

Preparation time: 15 minutes

Cooking time: 30 minutes

Servings: 1

Ingredients:

350g penne

2 x 212g tins cherry salmon, drained

1 lemon, zested and juiced

190g jar green pesto

250g package cherry tomatoes halved

100g bunch spring onions, finely chopped

125g package reduced-fat mozzarella

Directions:

Pre heat the oven to 220°C, buff 200°C. Boil the pasta for 5 minutes.

Drain reserving 100 ml drinking water.

Mix the salmon, lemon zest, and juice, then pesto, berries and half of the spring onions; season.

Mix the pasta and reserved cooking water to the dish. Mix the allowed pesto using 1 tablespoon water and then drizzle on the pasta.

Gently with mozzarella, top it with the rest of the spring onions and bake for 25 minutes until golden.

Nutrition:

Calories: 281

Total Fat: 25 g

Total Carbohydrates: 72 g

Protein: 43 g

Day 60. Sri Lankan-Style Sweet Potato Curry

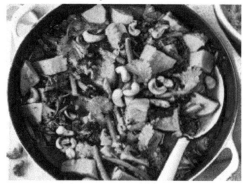

Preparation time: 25 minutes

Cooking time: 40 minutes

Servings: 1

Ingredients:

1/2 onion, roughly sliced

3 garlic cloves, roughly sliced

25g sliced ginger, chopped and peeled

15g fresh coriander stalks and leaves split leaves sliced

2 1/2 tablespoon moderate tikka curry powder

60g package cashew nuts

1 tablespoon olive oil

500g Red mere Farms sweet potatoes, peeled and cut into 3cm balls

400ml tin Isle Sun Coconut-milk

1/2 vegetable stock block, created as much as 300ml

200g Grower's Harvest long-grain rice

300g frozen green beans

150g Red mere Farms lettuce

1 Sun trail Farms lemon, 1/2 juiced, 1/2 cut into wedges to function

Directions:

Set the onion, ginger, garlic, coriander stalks tikka powder along with half of the cashew nuts in a food processor. Insert 2 tablespoons water and blitz to a chunky paste.

At a large skillet, warm the oil over moderate heat. Insert the paste and cook, stirring for 5 minutes. Bring the sweet potatoes, stir, and then pour into the coconut milk and stock. Bring to the simmer and boil for 25-35 minutes before the sweet potatoes are tender.

Meanwhile, cook the rice pack directions. Toast the rest of the cashews at a dry skillet.

Stir the beans into the curry and then simmer for 2 minutes. Insert the lettuce in handfuls, allowing each to simmer before adding the following; simmer for 1 minute.

Bring the lemon juice, to taste, & the majority of the coriander leaves. Scatter on the remaining coriander and cashews, then use the rice and lemon wedges.

Nutrition:

Calories: 747

Total Fat: 37 g

Total Carbohydrates: 90 g

Protein: 14 g

Day 61. Chicken Liver with Tomato Ragu

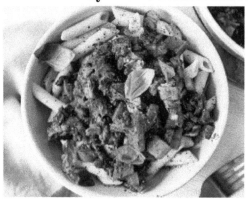

Preparation time: 15 minutes

Cooking time: 40 minutes

Servings: 4

Ingredients:

2 tablespoon olive oil

1 onion, finely chopped

2 carrots scrubbed and simmer

4 garlic cloves, finely chopped

1/4 x 30g pack fresh ginger, stalks finely chopped, leaves ripped

380g package poultry livers, finely chopped, and almost any sinew removed and lost

400g tin Grower's Harvest chopped berries

1 chicken stock cube, created around 300ml

1/2 tsp. caster sugar

300g penne

1/4 Sun trail Farms lemon, juiced

Directions:

On low-medium heat, put 1 tbsp. oil in a large skillet. Fry the onion and carrots to 10 minutes, stirring periodically.

Stir in the ginger and garlic pops and cook 2 minutes more. Transfer into a bowl set aside.

Twist the pan into high heat and then add the oil. Bring the chicken livers and simmer for 5 minutes until browned. Pour the onion mix to the pan and then stir in the tomatoes, sugar, and stock.

Season, bring to the boil, and then simmer for 20 minutes until reduced and thickened and also the liver is cooked through. Meanwhile, cook pasta.

Taste the ragu and put in a second pinch of sugar more seasoning, if needed. Put in a squeeze of lemon juice to taste and stir in two of the ripped basil leaves.

Divide the pasta between four bowls, then spoon across the ragu and top with the rest of the basil.

Nutrition:

Calories: 165

Total Fat: 5 g

Total Carbohydrates: 1 g

Protein: 25 g

Day 62. Minted Lamb with a Couscous Salad

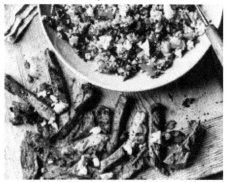

Preparation time: 15 minutes

Cooking time: 15 minutes

Servings: 1

Ingredients:

75g Couscous

1/2 chicken stock block, composed to 125ml

30g pack refreshing flat-leaf parsley, sliced

3 mint sprigs, leaves picked and sliced

1 tablespoon olive oil

200g pack suspended BBQ minted lamb leg beans, De-frosted

200g lettuce berries, sliced

1/4 tsp., sliced

1 spring onion, sliced

Pinch of ground cumin

1/2 lemon, zested and juiced

50g reduced-fat salad cheese

Directions:

Place the couscous into a heatproof bowl and then pour on the inventory. Cover and set aside for 10 minutes, then fluff with a fork and stir in the herbs.

Meanwhile, rub a little oil within the lamb steaks and season.

Mix the tomatoes, cucumber and spring onion into the couscous with the oil, the cumin, and lemon juice and zest. Crumble on the salad and serve with the bunny.

Nutrition:

Calories: 260

Total Fat: 15 g

Total Carbohydrates: 5 g

Protein: 25 g

Day 63. Jackfruit Tortilla Bowl

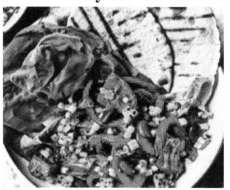

Preparation time: 5 minutes

Cooking time: 15 minutes

Servings: 2

Ingredients:

2 Sweet Corn cobettes

1 red chili, finely chopped

2 teaspoon olive oil

1 lime, juiced

15g fresh coriander, chopped, plus extra to garnish

150g package stained Jack Fruit in Texmex sauce

210g tin kidney beans, drained

125g roasted red peppers (in the jar), drained and chopped

2 whitened tortilla packs

1/2 round lettuce, ripped

Directions:

Heat a griddle Pan on a high temperature (or light a barbecue). Griddle that the cobettes to get 10 -12 minutes, turning until cooked and charred throughout. Remove from the pan and also stand upright onto a plank.

Use a sharp knife to carefully reduce the span of this corn, staying near to the heart, to clear away the kernels.

Mix that the kernels with the eucalyptus oil, half of the carrot juice along with half an hour of the coriander.

Heating the Jack fruit and sauce in a saucepan with the legumes, peppers, staying lime Coriander and juice on medium-low heating for 3 - 4 minutes until heated.

Griddle the wraps for 10 - 20 seconds each side to char. Tear into pieces and serve together with all the Jack Fruit lettuce and sweet corn salsa.

Nutrition:

Calories: 390

Total Fat: 8 g

Total Carbohydrates: 70 g

Protein: 13 g

Day 64. Super-Speedy Prawn Risotto

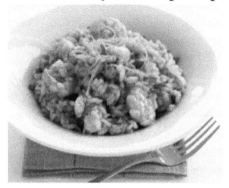

Preparation time: 10 minutes

Cooking time: 20 minutes

Servings: 4

Ingredients:

100g Diced Onion

2 X 250g packs whole-grain Rice & Quinoa

200g Frozen Garden Peas

2 x 150g packs Cooked and Peeled King Prawns

1/285g Tote water-cress

Directions:

Heating 1 tablespoon coconut oil in a skillet on medium-high heat and then put in 100g diced onion; cook for 5 minutes.

Insert 2 x 250g packs whole-grain Rice & Quinoa along with 175ml hot vegetable stock (or plain water); together side 200g suspended Garden Peas.

Gently split using rice using a wooden spoon. Cover and cook for 3 minutes, stirring occasionally, you can add two x 150g packs Cooked and Peeled King Prawns.

Cook for 12 minutes before prawns, peas, and rice have been piping hot, and the majority of the liquid was consumed.

Remove from heat. Chop 1/2 x 85g tote water-cress and stir throughout; up to taste. Top with watercress leaves and pepper to function.

Nutrition:

Calories: 347

Total Fat: 1.4 g

Cholesterol: 83 g

Sodium: 398 mg

Potassium: 322 mg

Total Carbohydrates: 63 g

Protein: 18 g

Day 65. Salmon Burgers

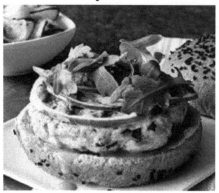

Preparation time: 20 minutes

Cooking time: 15 minutes

Servings: 5

Ingredients:

For Burgers:

1 teaspoon olive oil

1 cup fresh kale, tough ribs removed and chopped

1/3 cup shallots, chopped finely

Salt and ground black pepper, as required

16 ounces skinless salmon fillets

¾ cup cooked quinoa

2 tablespoons Dijon mustard

1 large egg, beaten

For Salad:

2½ tablespoons olive oil

2½ tablespoons red wine vinegar

Salt and ground black pepper, as required

8 cups fresh baby arugula

2 cups cherry tomatoes, halved

Directions:

For burgers:

In a large non-stick wok, heat the oil over medium heat and sauté the kale, shallot and kale, salt and black pepper for about 4-5 minutes.

Remove from heat and transfer the kale mixture into a large bowl. Set aside to cool slightly.

With a knife, chop 4 ounces of salmon and transfer into the bowl of kale mixture.

In a food processor, add the remaining salmon and pulse until finely chopped.

Transfer the finely chopped salmon into the bowl of kale mixture.

Then, add remaining ingredients and stir until fully combined.

Make 5 equal-sized patties from the mixture.

Heat a lightly greased large non-stick wok over medium heat and cook the patties for about 4-5 minutes per side.

For dressing:

In a glass bowl, add the oil, vinegar, shallots, salt and black pepper and beat until well combined.

Add arugula and tomatoes and toss to coat well.

Divide the salad onto on serving plates and top each with 1 patty.

Serve immediately.

Nutrition:

Calories: 329

Total Fat: 15.8 g

Saturated Fat: 2.4 g

Cholesterol: 77 mg

Sodium: 177 mg

Total Carbohydrates: 24 g

Fiber: 3.6 g

Sugar: 2.7 g

Protein: 24.9 g

Day 66. Tofu and Veggies Curry

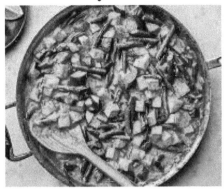

Preparation time: 20 minutes

Cooking time: 30 minutes

Servings: 1

Ingredients:

1 (16-ounce) block firm tofu, drained, pressed and cut into ½-inch cubes

2 tablespoons coconut oil

1 medium yellow onion, chopped

1½ tablespoons fresh ginger, minced

2 garlic cloves, minced

1 tablespoon curry powder

Salt and ground black pepper, as required

1 cup fresh mushrooms, sliced

1 cup carrots, peeled and sliced

1 (14-ounce) can unsweetened coconut milk

½ cup vegetable broth

2 teaspoons light brown sugar

10 ounces broccoli florets

1 tablespoon fresh lime juice

¼ cup fresh basil leaves, sliced thinly

Directions:

In a Dutch oven, heat the oil over medium heat and sauté the onion, ginger and garlic for about 5 minutes.

Stir in the curry powder, salt and black pepper and cook for about 2 minutes, stirring occasionally.

Add the mushrooms and carrot and cook for about 4-5 minutes.

Stir in the coconut milk, broth and brown sugar and bring to a boil.

Add the tofu and broccoli and simmer for about 12-15 minutes, stirring occasionally.

Stir in the lime juice and remove from the heat.

Serve hot.

Nutrition:

Calories: 184

Total Fat: 11.1 g

Saturated Fat: 6.9 g

Sodium: 55 mg

Total Carbohydrates: 14.3 g

Fiber: 4.5 g

Sugar: 5 g

Protein: 10.5 g

Day 67. Chicken with Veggies

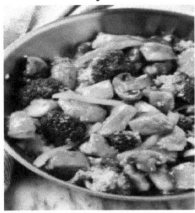

Preparation time: 15 minutes

Cooking time: 25 minutes

Servings: 1

Ingredients:

3 tablespoons olive oil

1 pound skinless, boneless chicken breast, cubed

1 medium onion, chopped

6 garlic cloves, minced

2 cups fresh mushrooms, sliced

16 ounces small broccoli florets

¼ cup water

Salt and ground black pepper, as required

Directions:

Heat the oil in a large wok over medium heat and cook the chicken cubes for about 4-5 minutes.

With a slotted spoon, transfer the chicken cubes onto a plate.

In the same wok, add the onion and sauté for about 4-5 minutes.

Add the mushrooms and cook for about 4-5 minutes.

Stir in the cooked chicken, broccoli and water, covered for about 8-10 minutes, stirring occasionally.

Stir in salt and black pepper and remove from heat.

Serve hot.

Nutrition:

Calories: 197

Total Fat: 10.1 g

Saturated Fat: 2 g

Cholesterol: 44 mg

Sodium: 82 mg

Total Carbohydrates: 8.5 g

Fiber: 2.7 g

Sugar: 2.5 g

Protein: 20.1 g

Day 68. Steak with Veggies

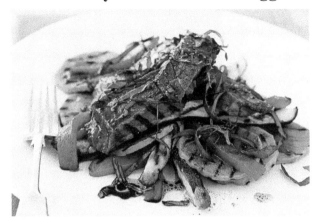

Preparation time: 15 minutes

Cooking time: 12 minutes

Servings: 4

Ingredients:

2 tablespoons coconut oil

4 garlic cloves, minced

1 pound beef sirloin steak, cut into bite-sized pieces

Ground black pepper, as required

1½ cups carrots, peeled and cut into matchsticks

1½ cups fresh kale, tough ribs removed and chopped

3 tablespoons tamari

Directions:

Melt the coconut oil in a wok over medium heat and sauté the garlic for about 1 minute.

Add the beef and black pepper and stir to combine.

Increase the heat to medium-high and cook for about 3-4 minutes or until browned from all sides.

Add the carrot, kale and tamari and cook for about 4-5 minutes.

Remove from the heat and serve hot.

Nutrition:

Calories: 311

Total Fat: 13.8 g

Saturated Fat: 8.6 g

Cholesterol: 101 mg

Sodium: 700 mg

Total Carbohydrates: 8.4 g

Fiber: 1.6 g

Sugar: 2.3 g

Protein: 37.1 g

Day 69. Parsley Lamb Chops with Kale

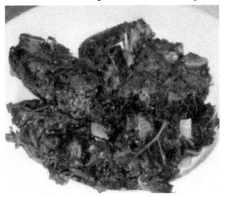

Preparation time: 25 minutes

Cooking time: 11 minutes

Servings: 4

Ingredients:

1 garlic clove, minced

1 tablespoon fresh parsley leaves, minced

Salt and ground black pepper, as required

4 lamb loin chops

4 cups fresh baby kale

Directions:

Pre heat the grill to high heat. Grease the grill grate.

In a bowl, add garlic, rosemary, salt and black pepper and mix well.

Coat the lamb chops with the herb mixture generously.

Place the chops onto the hot side of grill and cook for about 2 minutes per side.

Now, move the chops onto the cooler side of the grill and cook for about 6-7 minutes.

Divide the kale onto serving plates and top each with 1 chop and serve.

Nutrition:

Calories: 301

Total Fat: 10.5 g

Saturated Fat: 3.8 g

Cholesterol: 128 mg

Sodium: 176 mg

Total Carbohydrates: 7.8 g

Fiber: 1.4 g

Protein: 41.9 g

Day 70. Shrimp with Veggies

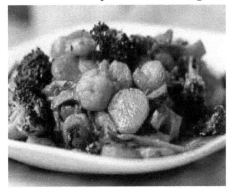

Preparation time: 15 minutes

Cooking time: 8 minutes

Servings: 5

Ingredients:

For Sauce

1 tablespoon fresh ginger, grated

2 garlic cloves, minced

3 tablespoons low-sodium soy sauce

1 tablespoon red wine vinegar

1 teaspoon brown sugar

¼ teaspoon red pepper flakes, crushed

For Shrimp Mixture

3 tablespoons olive oil

1½ pounds medium shrimp, peeled and deveined

12 ounces broccoli florets

8 ounces, carrot, peeled and sliced

Directions:

For sauce:

In a bow, place all the ingredients and beat until well combined. Set aside.

In a large wok, heat oil over medium-high heat and cook the shrimp for about 2 minutes, stirring occasionally.

Add the broccoli and carrot and cook about 3-4 minutes, stirring frequently.

Stir in the sauce mixture and cook for about 1-2 minutes.

Serve immediately.

Nutrition:

Calories: 298

Total Fat: 10.7 g

Saturated Fat: 1.3 g

Cholesterol: 305 mg

Sodium: 882 mg

Total Carbohydrates: 7 g

Fiber: 2g

Sugar: 2.4 g

Protein: 45.5 g

Day 71. Chickpeas with Swiss chard

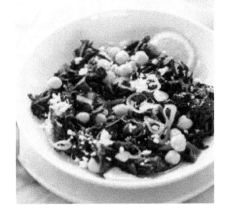

Preparation time: 15 minutes

Cooking time: 12 minutes

Servings: 4

Ingredients:

2 tablespoon olive oil

2 garlic cloves, sliced thinly

1 large tomato, chopped finely

2 bunches fresh Swiss chard, trimmed

1 (18-ounce) can chickpeas, drained and rinsed

Salt and ground black pepper, as required

¼ cup water

1 tablespoon fresh lemon juice

2 tablespoons fresh parsley, chopped

Directions:

Heat the oil in a large nonstick wok over medium heat and sauté the garlic for about 1 minute.

Add the tomato and cook for about 2-3 minutes, crushing with the back f spoon.

Stir in remaining ingredients except lemon juice and parsley and cook for about 5-7 minutes.

Drizzle with the lemon juice and remove from the heat.

Serve hot with the garnishing of parsley.

Nutrition:

Calories: 217

Total Fat: 8.3 g

Sodium: 171 mg

Total Carbohydrates: 26.2 g

Fiber: 6.6 g

Sugar: 1.8 g

Protein: 8.8 g

Day 72. Chicken & Berries Salad

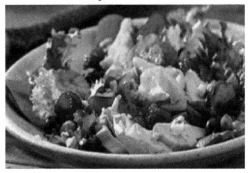

Preparation time: 20 minutes

Cooking time: 16 minutes

Servings: 8

Ingredients:

2 pounds boneless, skinless chicken breasts

½ cup olive oil

¼ cup fresh lemon juice

2 tablespoons maple syrup

1 garlic clove, minced

Salt and ground black pepper, as required

2 cups fresh strawberries, hulled and sliced

2 cups fresh blueberries

10 cups fresh baby arugula

Directions:

For marinade: in a large bowl, add oil, lemon juice, Erythritol, garlic, salt and black pepper and beat until well combined.

In a large re-sealable plastic bag, place the chicken and ¾ cup of marinade.

Seal bag and shake to coat well.

Refrigerate overnight.

Cover the bowl of remaining marinade and refrigerate before serving.

Preheat the grill to medium heat. Grease the grill grate.

Remove the chicken from bag and discard the marinade.

Place the chicken onto grill grate and grill, covered for about 5-8 minutes per side.

Remove chicken from grill and cut into bite sized pieces.

In a large bowl, add the chicken pieces, strawberries and spinach and mix.

Place the reserved marinade and toss to coat.

Serve immediately.

Nutrition:

Calories: 377

Total Fat: 21.5 g

Cholesterol: 101 mg

Sodium: 126 mg

Total Carbohydrates: 12.6 g

Fiber: 2 g

Sugar: 9 g

Protein: 34.1 g

Day 73. Beef & Kale Salad

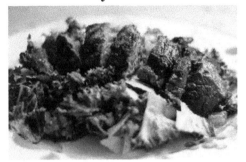

Preparation time: 15 minutes

Cooking time: 8 minutes

Servings: 2

Ingredients:

For Steak:

2 teaspoons olive oil

2 (4-ounce) strip steaks

Salt and ground black pepper, as required

For Salad:

¼ cup carrot, peeled and shredded

¼ cup cucumber, peeled, seeded and sliced

¼ cup radish, sliced

¼ cup cherry tomatoes, halved

3 cups fresh kale, tough ribs removed and chopped

For Dressing:

1 tablespoon extra-virgin olive oil

1 tablespoon fresh lemon juice

Salt and ground black pepper, as required

Directions:

For steak:

In a large heavy-bottomed wok, heat the oil over high heat and cook the steaks with salt and black pepper for about 3-4 minutes per side.

Transfer the steaks onto a cutting board for about 5 minutes before slicing.

For salad:

Place all ingredients in a salad bowl and mix.

For dressing:

Place all ingredients in another bowl and beat until well combined.

Cut the steaks into desired sized slices against the grain.

Place the salad onto each serving plate.

Top each plate with steak slices.

Drizzle with dressing and serve.

Nutrition:

Calories" 262

Total Fat: 12 g

Cholesterol: 63 mg

Sodium: 506 mg

Total Carbohydrates: 15.2 g

Fiber: 2.5g

Sugar: 3.3 g

Protein: 25.2 g

Day 74. Grilled Salmon Fillet with Chilies and Avocado Puree

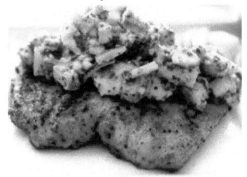

Preparation time: 10 minutes

Cooking time: 40 minutes

Servings: 3

Ingredients:

2 ripe avocados

2 tablespoons of lime juice

Salt

Pepper

4 fresh salmon fillets of 200 g each

For the chili sauce:

2 chilies

4 teaspoons of lime juice

4 teaspoons of honey

4 spoons of extra virgin olive oil

1 large shallot

Directions:

Cut the two avocados in half and remove the pulp with a teaspoon. Transfer it to the mixer with the lime juice and reduce everything in a silky and homogeneous cream. Salt rule and fresh reel pepper.

Prepare the sauce by cutting the peppers into rounds, removing the seeds. In a small bowl mix them with the sliced shallot, lime juice, honey and oil. Season with salt and mix well.

Cook the salmon fillets on a hot cast iron plate for about 4 minutes on the skin side. Turn them over, add a drizzle of oil and complete the cooking according to the thickness.

Season with salt and pepper, tassel the fillets with the chili sauce and serve immediately with the avocado puree.

Nutrition:

Calories: 170

Total Fat: 5 g

Cholesterol: 70 mg

Calcium: 20 mg

Protein: 25 g

Day 75. Salmon and Capers

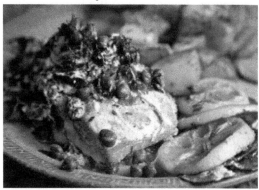

Preparation time: 5 minutes

Cooking time: 25 minutes

Servings: 2

Ingredients:

75g (3oz) Greek yogurt

4 salmon fillets, skin removed

4 teaspoons Dijon Mustard

1 tablespoon capers, chopped

2 teaspoons fresh parsley

Zest of 1 lemon

Directions:

In a bowl, mix together the yogurt, mustard, lemon zest, parsley and capers. Thoroughly coat the salmon in the mixture.

Place the salmon under a hot grill (broiler) and cook for 3-4 minutes on each side, or until the fish is cooked.

Serve with mashed potatoes and vegetables or a large green leafy salad.

Nutrition:

Calories: 400

Total Fat: 23 g

Cholesterol: 130 mg

Total Carbohydrates: 3 g

Protein: 40 g

Day 76. Asian Slaw

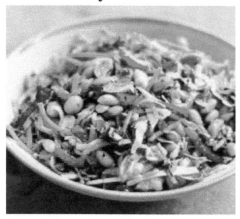

Preparation time: 5 minutes

Cooking time: 25 minutes

Servings: 2

Ingredients:

2 cups Red cabbage, shredded

2 cups Broccoli florets, chopped

1 cup Carrots, shredded

1 Red onion, finely sliced

1/2 Red bell pepper, finely sliced

1/2 Cilantro, chopped

1 tbsp. Sesame seeds

1/2 Peanuts, chopped

2 tsp. Sriracha

1/4 Rice wine vinegar

1/2 Sesame seed oil

1 tsp. Sea salt

1 clove Garlic, minced

2 tbsp. Peanut butter, natural

2 tbsp. extra virgin olive oil

2 tbsp. Tamari sauce

2 tsp. Ginger, peeled and grated

2 tsp. Honey

1/4 Black pepper, ground

Directions:

In a large salad bowl toss the vegetables, cilantro, and peanuts.

In a smaller bowl, whisk together the remaining ingredients until emulsified. Pour this dressing over the vegetables and toss together until fully coated.

Chill the slaw for at least ten minutes, so that the flavors meld. Refrigerate the Asian slaw for up to a day in advance for deeper flavors.

Nutrition:

Calories: 150

Total Fat: 5 g

Total Carbohydrates: 10 g

Protein: 2 g

Day 77. Egg Fried Buckwheat

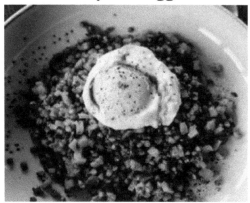

Preparation time: 5 minutes

Cooking time: 45 minutes

Servings: 2

Ingredients:

2 Eggs, beaten

2 tbsp. extra virgin olive oil

1 Onion, diced

1/2 Peas, frozen

2 Carrots, finely diced

2 cloves Garlic, minced

1 tsp. Ginger, grated

2 Green onions, thinly sliced

2 tbsp. Tamari sauce

2 tsp. Sriracha sauce

3 cups cooked buckwheat groats, cold

Directions:

Add half of the olive oil to a large skillet or set to medium heat then add the egg, stir constantly until it is fully cooked. Remove the egg and transfer it to another dish.

Add the remaining olive oil to your wok along with the peas, carrots, and onion. Cook until the carrots and onions are softened, about four minutes.

Add in the grated ginger and minced garlic, cooking for an additional minute until fragrant.

Add the sriracha sauce, tamari sauce, and cooked buckwheat groats to the wok. Continue to cook the buckwheat groats and stir the mixture until the buckwheat is warmed all the way through and the flavors have melded, about 2 minutes.

Add the cooked eggs and green onions to the wok, giving it a good toss to combine and serve warm.

Nutrition:

Calories: 430

Total Fat: 20 g

Total Carbohydrates: 30 g

Protein: 25 g

Day 78. Sautéed Red Cabbage

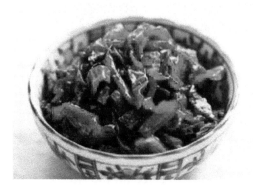

Preparation time: 5 minutes

Cooking time: 45 minutes

Servings: 2

Ingredients:

1 head small Red cabbage, thinly sliced

2 tablespoons extra virgin olive oil

1/2 Black pepper, ground

1 tbsp. Thyme, fresh, chopped

1/2 Apple cider vinegar

1 1/2 Sea salt

Directions:

When slicing your red cabbage into thin ribbons make sure to remove and discard the core.

Add the extra virgin olive oil to a large skillet with a heavy bottom over medium-high heat. Once warm, add in the red cabbage, sea salt, and pepper.

Sauté the cabbage until tender and start to brown, about 10 to 15 minutes. You don't need to constantly stir the cabbage, but give it a good stir once every few minutes. By doing this, you will allow the cabbage to caramelize without sticking.

Remove the cabbage from the heat and stir in the thyme and apple cider vinegar.

Taste the dish and adjust the seasonings to taste. You might want to even add an extra splash of apple cider vinegar if you will like a little more pop to the dish.

Nutrition:

Calories: 110

Total Fat: 1 g

Protein: 2 g

Day 79. Kale and Corn Succotash

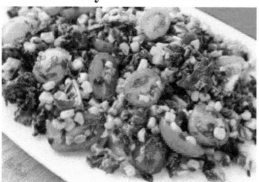

Preparation time: 5 minutes

Cooking time: 55 minutes

Servings: 2

Ingredients:

2 cups Corn kernels

1/2 Black pepper, ground

2 cups Kale, chopped

1 Red onion, finely diced

2 cloves Garlic, minced

1 cup Grape tomatoes, sliced in half lengthwise

1 teaspoon Sea salt

2 tablespoons Parsley, chopped

1 tablespoon extra-virgin olive oil

Directions:

Into a large skillet pour the olive oil, red onion, and the corn kernels, sautéing until hot and tender, about four minutes.

Add the sea salt, garlic, kale, and black pepper to the skillet, cooking until the kale has wilted, about three to five minutes.

Remove the large skillet from the stove and toss in the parsley and fresh grape tomatoes. Serve warm.

Nutrition:

Calories: 220

Total Fat: 11 g

Protein: 6 g

Day 80. Baked Vegetables

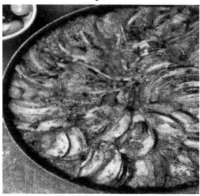

Preparation time: 5 minutes

Cooking time: 25 minutes

Servings: 2

Ingredients:

3 white onions

3 large fleshy tomatoes

4 spoons of stale breadcrumbs

Oregano

Extra virgin olive oil

Salt

4 large potatoes

Directions:

Prepare the vegetables in the oven by starting to peel and wash the potatoes.

Dry them and cut them into slices about one centimeter thick. Peel the onions and cut them into slices of the same thickness. Also wash and slice the tomatoes.

Brush a round baking pan with oil and arrange the vegetables in concentric circles alternating slices of potatoes, onions and tomatoes.

Sprinkle with breadcrumbs and oregano, season with a drizzle of oil and salt.

Bake at 170-180 ° for 30 minutes.

Withdraw vegetables in the oven, let them settle for about ten minutes and serve immediately on the table.

Nutrition:

Calories: 160

Total Fat: 5 g

Total Carbohydrates: 25 g

Protein: 3 g

Day 81. Peanut Broccoli Buckwheat Bowls

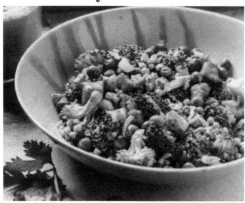

Preparation time: 5 minutes

Cooking time: 25 minutes

Servings: 2

Ingredients:

1 cup Buckwheat, uncooked

1 cup Frozen peas, thawed

14 ounces Tofu, extra-firm, pressed to remove excess liquid

24 ounces Broccoli florets

1 Red onion, diced

1/4 cup Parsley, chopped

1 1/2 Sea salt

2 cloves Garlic, minced

The Sauce:

1/4 Tamari sauce

1/2 Water

1/2 Peanut butter, natural sugar-free

3 tablespoons Lime juice

1 teaspoon Tahini paste

1/2 teaspoon Sriracha paste

1-inch nob Ginger root, peeled

2 cloves Garlic, minced

1/2 teaspoon Maple syrup

Directions:

Pour the water, tamari sauce, and other ingredients for the sauce into a blender and combine it on high speed until completely smooth.

Adjust the thickness to your taste, adding more water if desired. Taste and adjust the flavors to your preferences. Place the sauce to the side while you assemble the bowls.

Once you have drained the excess liquid off of the tofu (this is best done with a tofu press) slice the block in half lengthwise, so that you have two rectangular bricks. Slice both bricks of tofu into bite-sized cubes.

Set the sliced cubes of tofu on a baking sheet and toss them with half of the sea salt, baking them in an oven preheated to a temperature of Fahrenheit 400 degrees until crispy, about 25-30 minutes. Halfway through the cooking process flip the cubes over so that they crisp evenly.

Cook the buckwheat. Add the two cups of water into a pan and bring it to a boil before stirring in the remaining sea salt and the buckwheat grains.

Cover with a lid, reduce the heat to medium-low, and allow it to cook until the water is absorbed, about fifteen minutes.

While the tofu and buckwheat cooks begin preparing the vegetables. Chop the florets of broccoli into bite-size chunks and then add it into a large bowl along with the red onion and the prepared peanut sauce.

Toss together until the broccoli and onions is coated in the sauce then transfer the vegetables

Using a large fork fluff the cooked buckwheat and stir in the minced garlic. Divide the buckwheat between bowls for serving, top with the broccoli mixture, and lastly the tofu cubes. Enjoy while warm.

Nutrition:

Calories: 130

Total Fat: 7 g

Total Carbohydrates: 15 g

Protein: 2 g

Day 82. Roast Pork Beer with Onions

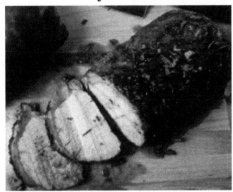

Preparation time: 5 minutes

Cooking time: 2 hours and 30 minutes

Servings: 1

Ingredients:

2 bay leaves

3 sprigs of thyme

300 ml of light beer

Extra virgin olive oil

30 g of butter

Salt

Black pepper

1 kg of loin or pork shoulder

800 g of blond onions

Directions:

To make the beer roast pork with onions, start tying the piece of meat with several turns of kitchen string.

Massage it with a pinch of salt and ground pepper, then brown it in a saucepan with the butter and 4 tablespoons of oil.

Turn it well on all sides so that the browning takes place uniformly. Take the roast from the saucepan and keep it warm.

Add the peeled and finely chopped onions, bay leaves and thyme sprigs to the cooking juices.

Mix well and let gently stew for 5 minutes. Then transfer the onions to an ovenproof dish, add the meat and drizzle everything with the beer.

Cover with a lid or aluminum foil and transfer the dish to the oven, preheated to 150 ° for 2 hours and 30 minutes.

After cooking, remove the aromatic herbs and transfer the pork roast to the beer with onions on a serving plate. Serve it sliced with its cooking sauce.

Nutrition:

Calories: 305

Total Fat: 21 g

Cholesterol: 80 mg

Sodium: 695 mg

Potassium: 300 mg

Total Carbohydrates: 7 g

Protein: 21 g

Day 83. Quinoa Nut and Radicchio Meatballs

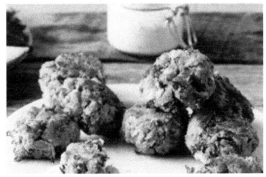

Preparation time: 10 minutes

Cooking time: 50 minutes

Servings: 8

Ingredients:

120 grams of white quinoa

2 tufts of late-growing radicchio di Treviso

80 grams of walnut kernels

2 teaspoons of turmeric

1 cup of foil flour

2 teaspoons of marjoram

Extra virgin olive oil

Salt and pepper to taste

Directions:

Wash the quinoa and boil it in lightly salted water until the seeds open and are soft.

When the quinoa is cooked, squeeze it well, then add the turmeric and pepper and keep it aside.

In a centrifuge add the nuts, salt, pepper and radicchio washed, blanched and dried well, and add a drizzle of oil.

Blend everything until a cream is obtained. Add the quinoa cream.

With floured hands, form balls from the dough and roll them into a mix of flour and chives.

Crush the meatballs at the ends. If the dough is too soft, leave it to rest for half an hour or thicken it with a little flour.

Place the meatballs on a sheet of baking paper sprinkled and bake at 180° for 20 minutes. Halfway through cooking, turn the meatballs to the other side.

Take them out of the oven and place them on an absorbent sheet to remove excess oil. Serve them hot.

Nutrition:

Calories: 240

Total Fat: 8 g

Cholesterol: 53 mg

Total Carbohydrates: 27 g

Protein: 17 g

Day 84. Chicken Paprika and Vegetables

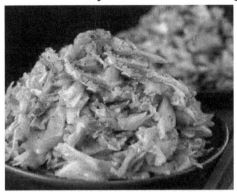

Preparation time: 15 minutes

Cooking time: 50 minutes

Servings: 4

Ingredients:

60 gr of extra virgin olive oil

40 grams of paprika

2 orange carrots

Half celeriac

3 turnips

Chicken wings 300 g

Vegetable broth 1 liter

Thyme and rosemary

Fresh bay 2 leaves

Pepper and salt to taste

Lemon

1 cup of chopped cabbage

Directions:

Clean and chop celeriac, turnip and carrot.

In a large pan, heat a drizzle of oil and add the chicken wings, paprika and chopped vegetables, cook for a few minutes.

Add salt and pepper, thyme and rosemary on the chicken wings and add a ladle of vegetable stock, cover the pan and let it boil.

When the broth dries add another ladle, and continue cooking the chicken on a low flame for about 40 minutes.

In the meantime, remove the outer leaves of the cabbage, wash it and chop it up, put it in the pan with the paprika chicken and continue to cook with the help of the stock until the cabbage is cooked.

Put out the fire, cover and let it rest for a few minutes before serving.

Nutrition:

Calories: 150

Total Fat: 2 g

Cholesterol: 68 mg

Total Carbohydrates: 4 g

Protein: 28 g

Day 85. Buckwheat Burger

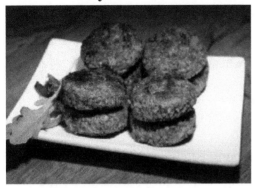

Preparation time: 15 minutes

Cooking time: 40 minutes

Servings: 3

Ingredients:

200 g Buckwheat without peel

Pound of red lentils

35 g Pumpkin seeds

4 tablespoons Baking powder

1/2 red onion, Tropia variety

1 slice Garlic

Oregano, thyme or other spices to taste

Rosemary

Soy sauce

Pepper

Yellow polenta flour

Directions:

Pour about 600 ml of water into a large pot.

Clean the onion and cut it thin, mince the garlic and wash the lentils. Put all the ingredients, including the spices, in the pot with water and add the buckwheat.

Light the fire and cook until all the water is absorbed. When cooking, add the rosemary sprig (which you will remove at the end)

When cooked, pour everything into a fairly large container, complete by combining the chopped pumpkin seeds and yeast, mix well and let everything cool. With your hands a little oiled, take a small amount of the mixture and form the burger. Pass them in the yellow polenta flour.

As you prepare them, place them on a baking tray, on which you will have placed the greaseproof baking paper, and bake at 180°. It's half cooked, turn them over and let them cook again. The cooking time is about twenty minutes.

Alternatively, burgers can cook in a pan with a drizzle of oil for fifteen minutes. Serve the burgers with some arugula.

Nutrition:

Calories: 185

Total Fat: 10 g

Total Carbohydrates: 25 g

Protein: 9 g

Day 86. Tofu and Buckwheat Salad

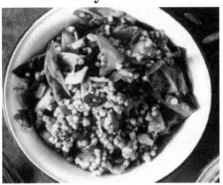

Preparation time: 10 minutes

Cooking time: 20 minutes

Servings: 4

Ingredients:

300 g Buckwheat

400 gr Cherry tomatoes

125 g Natural tofu

10 leaves of Basil

150 g Sunflower seeds

Extra virgin olive oil and Salt

Directions:

Prepare a pot almost full of cold water and put it on the stove.

Wash the buckwheat carefully under running water, pour it into the pot on the stove and let it cook for about 20 minutes.

In a large container put some basil leaves washed with care and the tomatoes washed and cut into four pieces.

Once cooked, drain the buckwheat and cool it under running water.

Cut the tofu into pieces and add it together with the wheat in the container with the tomatoes.

Add the remaining basil leaves and sunflower seeds, salt and pepper system and finally add a drizzle of oil, mix everything well and let it rest.

You can have the salad still warm and freshly made or leave it in the fridge and eat it cold.

Nutrition:

Calories: 400

Fat: 10 g

Carbohydrates: 50 g

Protein: 20 g

Day 87. Courgette Tortillas

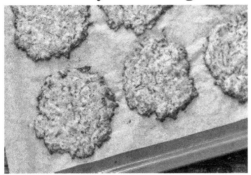

Preparation time: 5 minutes

Cooking time: 20 minutes

Servings: 4

Ingredients:

20 g Butter in chunks or alternatively 2 spoons of coconut oil

2 green zucchini

4 whole eggs

Pepper and salt to taste

Parsley or chives

Directions:

Wash and slice the zucchini.

In a high pot, melt the butter or heat the oil. When it is ready, pour in the freshly cut zucchini and stir well until they soften.

In a bowl break the four eggs, beat them adding salt, pepper, parsley or chives. Pour the mixture over the zucchini.

Cook until the eggs are almost cooked, before finishing put the pot in the oven and turn on the grill to toast the tortillas.

Nutrition:

Calories: 97

Fat: 1 g

Carbohydrates: 20 g

Protein: 4 g

Snacks and Desserts

88.Baby Spinach Snack

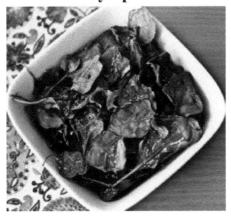

Preparation time: 10 minutes

Cooking time: 10 minutes

Servings: 1

Ingredients:

2 cups baby spinach, washed

A pinch of black pepper

½ tablespoon olive oil

½ teaspoon garlic powder

Directions:

Spread the baby spinach on a lined baking sheet, add oil, black pepper and garlic powder, toss a bit.

Bake at 350 degrees F for 10 minutes, divide into bowls and serve as a snack.

Enjoy!

Nutrition:

Calories: 125

Fat: 4 g

Fiber: 1 g

Carbohydrates: 4 g

Protein: 2 g

Day 88.   Sesame Dip

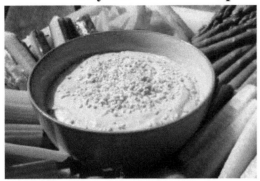

Preparation time: 10 minutes

Cooking time: 0 minutes

Servings: 1

Ingredients:

1 cup sesame seed paste, pure

Black pepper to the taste

1 cup veggie stock

½ cup lemon juice

½ teaspoon cumin, ground

3 garlic cloves, chopped

Directions:

In your food processor, mix the sesame paste with black pepper, stock, lemon juice, cumin and garlic.

Pulse very well, divide into bowls and serve as a party dip.

Enjoy!

Nutrition:

Calories: 120

Fat: 12 g

Fiber: 2 g

Carbohydrates: 7 g

Protein: 4 g

Day 89. Rosemary Squash Dip

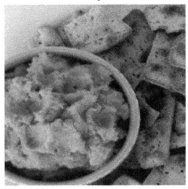

Preparation time: 10 minutes

Cooking time: 40 minutes

Servings: 1

Ingredients:

1 cup butternut squash, peeled and cubed

1 tablespoon water

Cooking spray

2 tablespoons coconut milk

2 teaspoons rosemary, dried

Black pepper to the taste

Directions:

Spread squash cubes on a lined baking sheet, spray some cooking oil, introduce in the oven, bake at 365 degrees F for 40 minutes.

Transfer to your blender, add water, milk, rosemary and black pepper, pulse well, divide into small bowls and serve.

Enjoy!

Nutrition:

Calories: 182

Fat: 5 g

Fiber: 7 g

Carbohydrates: 12 g

Protein: 5 g

Day 90. Bean Spread

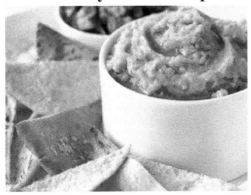

Preparation time: 10 minutes

Cooking time: 6 hours

Servings: 1

Ingredients:

1 cup white beans, dried

1 teaspoon apple cider vinegar

1 cup veggie stock

1 tablespoon water

Directions:

In your slow cooker, mix beans with stock, stir, cover, cook on Low for 6 hours.

Drain and transfer to your food processor, add vinegar and water, pulse well, divide into bowls and serve.

Enjoy!

Nutrition:

Calories: 181

Fat: 6 g

Fiber: 5 g

Carbohydrates: 9 g

Protein: 7 g

Day 91. Corn Spread

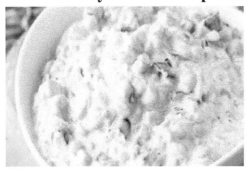

Preparation time: 10 minutes

Cooking time: 10 minutes

Servings: 1

Ingredients:

30 ounces canned corn, drained

2 green onions, chopped

½ cup coconut cream

1 jalapeno, chopped

½ teaspoon chili powder

Directions:

In a small pan, combine the corn with green onions, jalapeno and chili powder, stir, and bring to a simmer.

Cook over medium heat for 10 minutes, leave aside to cool down, add coconut cream, stir well, divide into small bowls and serve as a spread.

Enjoy!

Nutrition:

Calories: 192

Fat: 5

Fiber 10

Carbohydrates: 11 g

Protein: 8 g

Day 92. Mushroom Dip

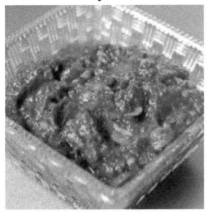

Preparation time: 10 minutes

Cooking time: 20 minutes

Servings: 1

Ingredients:

1 cup yellow onion, chopped

3 garlic cloves, minced

1 pound mushrooms, chopped

28 ounces tomato sauce, no-salt-added

Black pepper to the taste

Directions:

Put the onion in a pot, add garlic, mushrooms, black pepper and tomato sauce, and stir.

Cook over medium heat for 20 minutes, leave aside to cool down, divide into small bowls and serve.

Enjoy!

Nutrition:

Calories 215

Fat: 4 g

Fiber: 7 g

Carbohydrates: 3 g

Protein: 7 g

Day 93. Salsa Bean Dip

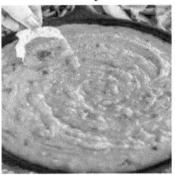

Preparation time: 10 minutes

Cooking time: 20 minutes

Servings: 1

Ingredients:

½ cup salsa

2 cups canned white beans, no-salt-added, drained and rinsed

1 cup low-fat cheddar, shredded

2 tablespoons green onions, chopped

Directions:

In a small pot, combine the beans with the green onions and salsa, stir, bring to a simmer over medium heat, and cook for 20 minutes

Add cheese, stir until it melts, and take off heat, leave aside to cool down, divide into bowls and serve.

Enjoy!

Nutrition:

Calories: 212

Fat: 5 g

Fiber: 6 g

Carbohydrates: 10 g

Protein: 8 g

Day 94. Mung Beans Snack Salad

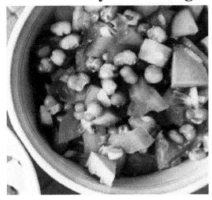

Preparation time: 10 minutes

Cooking time: 0 minutes

Servings: 1

Ingredients:

2 cups tomatoes, chopped

2 cups cucumber, chopped

3 cups mixed greens

2 cups mung beans, sprouted

2 cups clover sprouts

For the salad dressing:

1 tablespoon cumin, ground

1 cup dill, chopped

4 tablespoons lemon juice

1 avocado, pitted, peeled and roughly chopped

1 cucumber, roughly chopped

Directions:

In a salad bowl, mix tomatoes with 2 cups cucumber, greens, clover and mung sprout.

In your blender, mix cumin with dill, lemon juice, 1 cucumber and avocado, blend really well, add this to your salad, toss well and serve as a snack

Enjoy!

Nutrition:

Calories: 120

Fat: 0 g

Fiber: 2 g

Carbohydrates: 1 g

Protein: 6 g

Day 95. Greek Party Dip

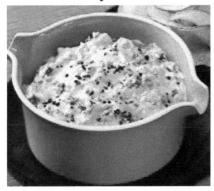

Preparation time: 10 minutes

Cooking time: 0 minutes

Servings: 1

Ingredients:

½ cup coconut cream

1 cup fat-free Greek yogurt

2 teaspoons dill, dried

2 teaspoons thyme, dried

1 teaspoon sweet paprika

2 teaspoons no-salt-added sun-dried tomatoes, chopped

2 teaspoons parsley, chopped

2 teaspoons chives, chopped

Black pepper to the taste

Directions:

In a bowl, mix cream with yogurt, dill with thyme, paprika, tomatoes, parsley, chives and pepper, stir well.

Divide into smaller bowls and serve as a dip.

Enjoy!

Nutrition:

Calories: 100

Fat: 1 g

Fiber: 4 g

Carbohydrates: 8 g

Protein: 3 g

Day 96. Zucchini Bowls

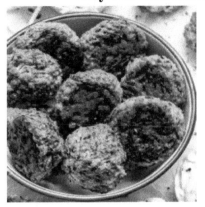

Preparation time: 10 minutes

Cooking time: 20 minutes

Servings: 12

Ingredients:

Cooking spray

½ cup dill, chopped

1 egg

½ cup whole wheat flour

Black pepper to the taste

1 yellow onion, chopped

2 garlic cloves, minced

3 zucchinis, grated

Directions:

In a bowl, mix zucchinis with garlic, onion, flour, pepper, egg and dill, stir well, shape small bowls out of this mix.

Arrange them on a lined baking sheet; grease them with some cooking spray.

Bake at 400 degrees F for 20 minutes, flipping them halfway, divide them into bowls and serve as a snack.

Enjoy!

Nutrition:

Calories: 120

Fat: 1 g

Fiber: 4 g

Carbohydrates: 12 g

Protein: 6 g

Day 97. Baking Powder Biscuits

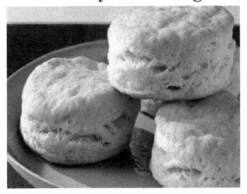

Preparation time: 10 minutes

Cooking time: 10 minutes

Servings: 1 2

Ingredients:

1 egg white

1 c. white whole-wheat flour

4 tbsp. of Non-hydrogenated vegetable shortening

1 tbsp. sugar

2/3 c. low-fat milk

1 c. unbleached all-purpose flour

4 tsps. Sodium-free baking powder

Directions:

Preheat oven to 450°F. Take out a baking sheet and set aside.

Place the flour, sugar, and baking powder into a mixing bowl and whisk well to combine.

Cut the shortening into the mixture using your fingers, and work until it resembles coarse crumbs. Add the egg white and milk and stir to combine.

Turn the dough out onto a lightly floured surface and knead 1 minute. Roll dough to ¾ inch thickness and cut into 12 rounds.

Place rounds on the baking sheet. Place baking sheet on middle rack in oven and bake 10 minutes.

Remove baking sheet and place biscuits on a wire rack to cool.

Nutrition:

Calories: 118

Fat: 4 g

Carbohydrates: 16 g

Protein: 3 g

Sugars: 0.2 g

Sodium: 294 mg

Day 98. Vegan Rice Pudding

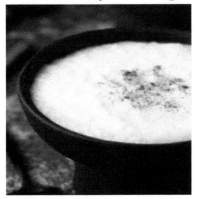

Preparation time: 5 minutes

Cooking time: 20 minutes

Servings: 8

Ingredients:

½ tsp. ground cinnamon

1 c. rinsed basmati

1/8 tsp. ground cardamom

¼ c. sugar

1/8 tsp. pure almond extract

1 quart vanilla nondairy milk

1 tsp. pure vanilla extract

Directions:

Measure all of the ingredients into a saucepan and stir well to combine. Bring to a boil over medium-high heat.

Once boiling, reduce heat to low and simmer, stirring very frequently, about 15–20 minutes.

Remove from heat and cool. Serve sprinkled with additional ground cinnamon if desired.

Nutrition:

Calories: 148

Fat: 2 g

Carbohydrates: 26 g

Protein: 4 g

Sugars: 35 g

Sodium: 150 mg

Day 99. Orange and Carrots

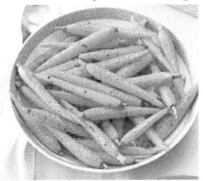

Preparation time: 5 minutes

Cooking time: 25 minutes

Servings: 1

Ingredients:

1 pound carrots, peeled and roughly sliced

1 yellow onion, chopped

1 tablespoon olive oil

Zest of 1 orange, grated

Juice of 1 orange

1 orange, peeled and cut into segments

1 tablespoon rosemary, chopped

A pinch of salt and black pepper

Directions:

Heat up a pan with the oil over medium-high heat.

Add the onion and sauté for 5 minutes.

Add the carrots, the orange zest and the other ingredients.

Cook over medium heat for 20 minutes more, divide between plates and serve.

Nutrition:

Calories: 140

Fat: 3.9 g

Fiber: 5 g

Carbohydrates: 26.1 g

Protein: 2.1 g

Day 100. Baked Broccoli and Pine Nuts

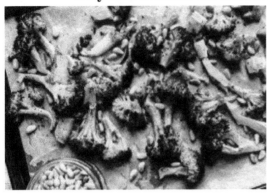

Preparation time: 10 minutes

Cooking time: 30 minutes

Servings: 1

Ingredients:

2 tablespoons olive oil

1 pound broccoli florets

1 tablespoon garlic, minced

1 tablespoon pine nuts, toasted

1 tablespoon lemon juice

2 teaspoons mustard

A pinch of salt and black pepper

Directions:

In a roasting pan, combine the broccoli with the oil, the garlic and the other ingredients, toss and bake at 380 degrees F for 30 minutes.

Divide everything between plates and serve as snack.

Nutrition:

Calories: 220

Fat: 6 g

Fiber: 2 g

Carbohydrates: 7 g

Protein: 6 g

Day 101. Turmeric Carrots

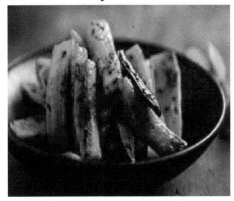

Preparation time: 10 minutes

Cooking time: 40 minutes

Servings: 1

Ingredients:

1 pound baby carrots, peeled

1 tablespoon olive oil

2 spring onions, chopped

2 tablespoons balsamic vinegar

2 garlic cloves, minced

1 teaspoon turmeric powder

1 tablespoon chives, chopped

¼ teaspoon cayenne pepper

A pinch of salt and black pepper

Directions:

Spread the carrots on a baking sheet lined with parchment paper, add the oil, the spring onions and the other ingredients, toss and bake at 380 degrees F for 40 minutes.

Divide the carrots between plates and serve.

Nutrition:

Calories: 79

Fat: 3.8 g

Fiber: 3.7 g

Carbohydrates: 10.9 g

Protein: 1 g

Day 102. Hawaii Salad

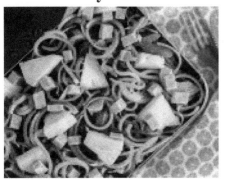

Preparation time: 10 minutes

Cooking time: 15 minutes

Servings: 1

Ingredients:

1 hand Arugula

1/2 pieces Red onion

1 piece winter carrot

2 pieces Pineapple slices

80 g Diced ham

1 pinch Salt

1 pinch Black pepper

Directions:

Cut the red onion into thin half rings.

Remove the peel and hard core from the pineapple and cut the pulp into thin pieces.

Clean the carrot and use a spiralizer to make strings.

Mix rocket and carrot in a bowl. Spread this over a plate.

Spread the red onion, pineapple and diced ham over the rocket.

Drizzle olive oil and balsamic vinegar on the salad to your taste.

Season it with salt and pepper.

Nutrition:

Calories: 150

Total Fat: 2.8 g

Cholesterol: 2 mg

Sodium: 42 mg

Potassium: 172 mg

Carbohydrates: 23 g

Protein: 2 g

Day 103. Fresh Salad with Orange Dressing

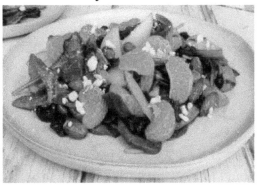

Preparation time: 10 minutes

Cooking time: 15 minutes

Servings: 1

Ingredients:

1 / 2 fruit Salad

1 piece yellow bell pepper

1 piece Red pepper

100 g Carrot (grated)

1 hand Almonds

Dressing:

4 tablespoon Olive oil

110 ml Orange juice (fresh)

1 tablespoon Apple cider vinegar

Directions:

Clean the peppers and cut them into long thin strips.

Tear off the lettuce leaves and cut them into smaller pieces.

Mix the salad with the peppers and the carrots processed in a bowl.

Roughly chop the almonds and sprinkle over the salad.

Mix all the ingredients for the dressing in a bowl.

Pour the dressing over the salad just before serving.

Nutrition:

Calories: 46.6

Total Fat: 0.1 g

Sodium: 230.8 mg

Potassium: 35.6 mg

Total Carbohydrates: 5.6 g

Protein: 0.7 g

Day 104. Sweet Potato Hash Brown

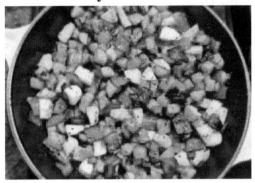

Preparation time: 5 minutes

Cooking time: 15 minutes

Servings: 2

Ingredients:

1 pinch Celtic sea salt

1 tablespoon Coconut oil

2 pieces Sweet potato

2 pieces Red onion

2 teaspoons Balsamic vinegar

1 piece Apple

125 g lean bacon strips

Directions:

Clean the red onions and cut them into half rings.

Heat a pan with a little coconut oil over medium heat. Fry the onion until it's almost done.

Add the balsamic vinegar and a pinch of salt and cook until the balsamic vinegar has boiled down. Put aside.

Peel the sweet potatoes and cut them into approx. 1.5 cm cubes.

Heat the coconut oil in a pan and fry the sweet potato cubes for 10 minutes.

Add the bacon strips for the last 2 minutes and fry them until you're done.

Cut the apple into cubes and add to the sweet potato cubes. Let it roast for a few minutes.

Then add the red onion and stir well.

Spread the sweet potato hash browns on 2 plates.

Nutrition:

Calories: 101

Total Fat: 7 g

Sodium: 5 mg

Potassium: 97 mg

Carbohydrates: 9 g

Protein: 0.8 g

Day 105. Herby French Fries with Herbs and Avocado Dip

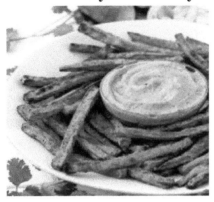

Preparation time: 15 minutes

Cooking time: 35 minutes

Servings: 1

Ingredient:

For the Fries:

1 / 2 pieces Celery

150 g Sweet potato

1 teaspoon dried oregano

1 / 2 teaspoon Dried basil

1 / 2 teaspoon Celtic sea salt

1 teaspoon Black pepper

1 1 / 2 tablespoon Coconut oil (melted)

Baking paper sheet

For the avocado dip:

1 piece Avocado

4 tablespoons Olive oil

1 tablespoon Mustard

1 teaspoon Apple cider vinegar

1 tablespoon Honey

2 cloves Garlic (pressed)

1 teaspoon dried oregano

Directions:

Preheat the oven to 205 ° C.

Peel the celery and sweet potatoes.

Cut the celery and sweet potatoes into (thin) French fries.

Place the French fries in a large bowl and mix with the coconut oil and herbs.

Shake the bowl a few times so that the fries are covered with a layer of the oil and herb mixture.

Place the chips in a layer on a baking sheet lined with baking paper or on a grill rack.

Bake for 25-35 minutes (turn over after half the time) until they have a nice golden brown color and are crispy.

For the avocado dip:

Puree all ingredients evenly with a hand blender or blender.

Nutrition:

Calories: 459

Total Fat: 27 g

Total Carbohydrates: 50 g

Protein: 4 g

Day 106. Spiced Burger

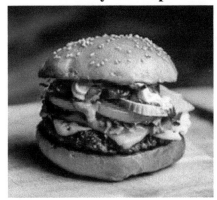

Preparation time: 20 minutes

Cooking time: 30 minutes

Serving: 1

Ingredients:

Ground beef 250 g

1 clove Garlic

1 teaspoon dried oregano

1 teaspoon Paprika powder

1 / 2 tsp. Caraway ground

Ingredients toppings:

4 pieces Mushrooms

1 piece Little Gem

1/4 pieces Zucchini

1/2 pieces Red onion

1 piece Tomato

Directions:

Squeeze the clove of garlic.

Mix all the ingredients for the burgers in a bowl. Divide the mixture into two halves and crush the halves into hamburgers.

Place the burgers on a plate and put in the fridge for a while.

Cut the zucchini diagonally into 1 cm slices.

Cut the red onion into half rings. Cut the tomato into thin slices and cut the leaves of the Little Gem salad.

Grill the hamburgers on the grill until they're done.

Place the mushrooms next to the burgers and grill on both sides until cooked but firm.

Place the zucchini slices next to it and grill briefly.

Now it's time to build the burger: Place 2 mushrooms on a plate then stack the lettuce, a few slices of zucchini and tomatoes. Then put the burger on top and finally add the red onion.

Nutrition:

Calories: 158

Fat: 8 g

Total Carbohydrates: 17 g

Protein: 3 g

Day 107. Ganache Squares

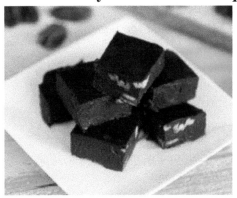

Preparation time: 15 minutes

Cooking time: 2 hours and 20 minutes

Servings: 10

Ingredients:

250 ml Coconut milk (can)

1 1/2 tablespoon Coconut oil

100 g Honey

1/2 teaspoon Vanilla extract

350 g pure chocolate (70% cocoa)

1 pinch Salt

2 hands Pecans

Directions:

Place the coconut milk in a saucepan and heat for 5 minutes over medium heat.

Add the vanilla extract, coconut oil and honey and cook for 15 minutes. Add a pinch of salt and stir well.

Break the chocolate into a bowl and pour the hot coconut milk over it. Keep stirring until all of the chocolate has dissolved in the coconut milk.

In the meantime, roughly chop the pecans. Heat a pan without oil and roast the pecans.

Stir the pecans through the ganache.

Let the ganache cool to room temperature. (You may be able to speed this up by placing the bowl in a bowl of cold water.)

Line a baking tin with a sheet of parchment paper. Pour the cooled ganache into it.

Place the ganache in the refrigerator for 2 hours to allow it to harden.

When the ganache has hardened, you can take it out of the mold and cut it into the desired shape.

Nutrition:

Calories: 141

Fat: 11 g

Carbohydrates: 9 g

Protein: 1 g

Day 108. Date Candy

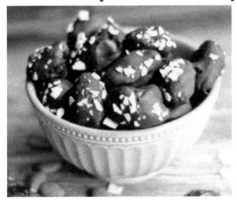

Preparation time: 20 minutes

Cooking time: 3 – 4 hours

Servings: 10

Ingredients:

10 pieces Medjool dates

1 hand Almonds

100 g pure chocolate (70% cocoa)

2 1/2 tablespoon Grated coconut

Directions:

Melt chocolate in a water bath.

Roughly chop the almonds.

In the meantime, cut the dates lengthways and take out the core.

Fill the resulting cavity with the roughly chopped almonds and close the dates again.

Place the dates on a sheet of parchment paper and pour the melted chocolate over each date.

Sprinkle the grated coconut over the chocolate dates.

Place the dates in the fridge so the chocolate can harden.

Day 109. Paleo Bars with Dates and Nuts

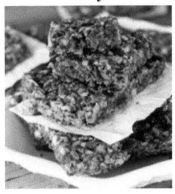

Preparation time: 10 minutes

Cooking time: 15 minutes

Servings: 16

Ingredients:

180 g Dates

60 g Almonds

60 g Walnuts

50 g Grated coconut

1 teaspoon Cinnamon

Directions:

Roughly chop the dates and soak them in warm water for 15 minutes.

In the meantime, roughly chop the almonds and walnuts.

Drain the dates.

Place the dates with the nuts, coconut and cinnamon in the food processor and mix to an even mass. (But not too long, crispy pieces or nuts make it particularly tasty)

Roll out the mass on 2 baking trays to form an approximately 1 cm thick rectangle.

Cut the rectangle into bars and keep each bar in a piece of parchment paper.

Nutrition:

Calories: 227

Total Fat: 19 g

Sodium: 9 mg

Carbohydrates: 12 g

Protein: 5 g

Day 110. Hazelnut Balls

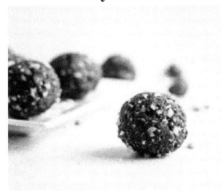

Preparation time: 20 minutes

Cooking time: 4 – 5 hours

Servings: 10

Ingredients:

130 g Dates

140 g Hazelnuts

2 tablespoon Cocoa powder

1/2 teaspoon Vanilla extract

1 teaspoon Honey

Directions:

Put the hazelnuts in a food processor and grind them until you get hazelnut flour (you can also use ready-made hazelnut flour).

Put the hazelnut flour in a bowl and set aside.

Put the dates in the food processor and grind them until you get a ball.

Add the hazelnut flour, vanilla extract, cocoa and honey and pulse until you get a nice and even mix.

Remove the mixture from the food processor and turn it into beautiful balls.

Store the balls in the fridge.

Nutrition:

Calories: 73

Total Fat: 5 g

Total Carbohydrates: 5 g

Protein: 1 g

Day 111. Pine and Sunflower Seed Rolls

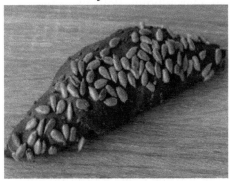

Preparation time: 20 minutes

Cooking time: 35 minutes

Servings: 10

Ingredients:

120 g Tapioca flour

1 teaspoon Celtic sea salt

4 tablespoon Coconut flour

120 ml Olive oil

120 ml Water (warm)

1 piece Egg (beaten)

150 g Pine nuts (roasted)

150 g Sunflower seeds (roasted)

Baking paper sheet

Directions:

Preheat the oven to 160 ° C.

Put the pine nuts and sunflower seeds in a small bowl and set aside.

Mix the tapioca with the salt and tablespoons of coconut flour in a large bowl. Pour the olive oil and warm water into the mixture.

Add the egg and mix until you get an even texture. If the dough is too thin, add 1 tablespoon of coconut flour at a time until it has the desired consistency.

Wait a few minutes between each addition of the flour so that it can absorb the moisture. The dough should be soft and sticky.

With a wet tablespoon, take tablespoons of batter to make a roll. Put some tapioca flour on your hands so the dough doesn't stick. Fold the dough with your fingertips instead of rolling it in your palms.

Place the roll in the bowl of pine nuts and sunflower seeds and roll it around until covered.

Line a baking sheet with parchment paper. Place the buns on the baking sheet.

Bake in the preheated oven for 35 minutes and serve warm.

Nutrition:

Calories: 163

Total Fat: 14 g

Fiber: 3 g

Total Carbohydrates: 6.5 g

Protein: 5 g

Day 112. Banana Dessert

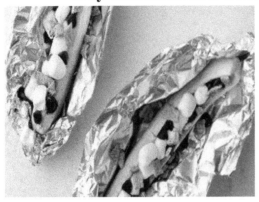

Preparation time: 5 minutes

Cooking time: 4 minutes

Servings: 2

Ingredients:

2 pieces Banana (ripe)

2 tablespoons pure chocolate (70% cocoa)

2 tablespoons Almond leaves

Directions:

Chop the chocolate finely, cut the banana lengthwise, but not completely, as the banana must serve as a casing for the chocolate.

Slightly slide on the banana, spread the finely chopped chocolate and almonds over the bananas.

Fold a kind of boat out of the aluminum foil that supports the banana well, with the cut in the banana facing up.

Place the two packets and grill them for about 4 minutes until the skin is dark.

Nutrition:

Calories: 105

Total Fat: 0.4 g

Sodium: 1.2 mg

Total Carbohydrates: 27 g

Protein: 1.3 g

Fiber: 3 g

Day 113. Strawberry Popsicles with Chocolate Dip

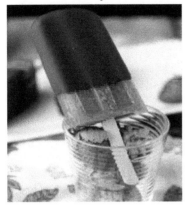

Preparation time: 20 minutes

Cooking time: 5 – 6 hours

Servings: 4

Ingredients:

125 g Strawberries

80 ml Water

100 g pure chocolate (70% cocoa)

Directions:

Clean the strawberries and cut them into pieces. Puree the strawberries with the water.

Pour the mixture into the Popsicle mold and put it in a skewer.

Place the molds in the freezer so the popsicles can freeze hard.

Once the popsicles are frozen hard, you can melt the chocolate in a water bath.

Dip the popsicles in the melted chocolate mixture.

Nutrition:

Calories: 60

Fiber: 1 g

Sugars: 14 g

Total Carbohydrates: 15 g

Day 114. Strawberry and Coconut Ice Cream

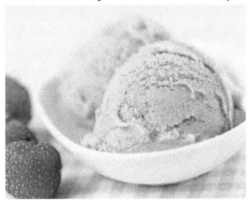

Preparation time: 20 minutes

Cooking time: 1 hour

Servings: 1

Ingredients:

400 ml Coconut milk (can)

1 hand Strawberries

1/2 pieces Lime

3 tablespoons Honey

Directions:

Clean the strawberries and cut them into large pieces.

Grate the lime, 1 teaspoon of lime peel is required. Squeeze the lime.

Put all ingredients in a blender and puree everything evenly.

Pour the mixture into a bowl and put it in the freezer for 1 hour.

Take the mixture out of the freezer and put it in the blender. Mix them well again.

Pour the mixture back into the bowl and freeze it until it is hard.

Before serving; take it out of the freezer about 10 minutes before scooping out the balls.

Nutrition:

Calories: 200

Total Fat: 11 g

Cholesterol: 0 mg

Sodium: 5 mg

Total Carbohydrates: 23 g

Protein: 1 g

Day 115. Coffee Ice Cream

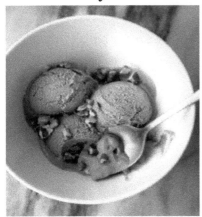

Preparation time: 15 minutes

Cooking time: 1 hour

Servings: 1

Ingredients:

180 ml Coffee

8 pieces Medjool dates

400 ml Coconut milk (can)

1 teaspoon Vanilla extract

Directions:

Make sure that the coffee has cooled down before using it.

Cut the dates into rough pieces.

Place the dates and coffee in a food processor and mix to an even mass.

Add coconut milk and vanilla and puree evenly.

Pour the mixture into a bowl and put it in the freezer for 1 hour.

Take the mixture out of the freezer and scoop it into the blender.

Pour it back into the bowl and freeze it until it's hard.

When serving; take it out of the freezer a few minutes before scooping ice cream balls with a spoon.

Nutrition:

Calories: 140

Total Fat: 7 g

Cholesterol: 25 mg

Sodium: 35 mg

Carbohydrates: 16 g

Day 116. Banana Strawberry Milkshake

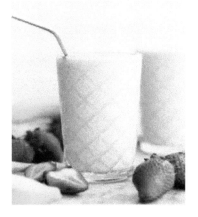

Preparation time: 10 minutes

Cooking time: 10 minutes

Servings: 1

Ingredients:

2 pieces Banana (frozen)

1 hand Strawberries (frozen)

250 ml Coconut milk (can)

Preparation:

Peel the bananas, slice them and place them in a bag or on a tray. Put them in the freezer the night before.

Put all ingredients in the blender and mix to an even milkshake.

Spread on the glasses.

Nutrition:

Calories: 110

Total Fat: 1 g

Cholesterol: 5 mg

Sodium: 40 mg

Carbohydrates: 23 g

Sugar: 16 g

Protein: 4 g

30 Day Meal Plan

The Sirtfood Diet contains two stages that last for a total of 3 weeks. From then on, you're able to carry on "sirtifying" your daily diet by adding many Sirtfoods as you possibly can to your daily meals.

It should be noted that the majority of the components and Sirtfoods are easy to find. A big part of the diet plan is its specialized green juice, which you must produce yourself daily.

Phase One

The very first phase lasts seven days, and also involves calorie limitation and a lot of green juice. It's meant to jumpstart your weight-loss reduction and promises to help you to lose 5 pounds in 7 days.

In the first three days of phase one, your calorie intake is confined to 1000 calories: You need to have three green juices every day and eat one meal made up of Sirtfoods.

On days 4-7, calories are raised to 1,500. This consists of two green juices every day and two Sirtfood-rich meals.

Phase Two

Phase Two goes on for two or three weeks. Throughout this "maintenance" period, you should gradually continue to lose weight.

There is no particular calorie limitation. As an alternative, you may eat three meals high in Sirtfoods and one green juice daily.

After the Diet

After you finish the diet, you will repeat both of these stages as frequently as desired for additional weight reduction.

You are encouraged to keep on your daily diet after completing those periods by incorporating Sirtfoods consistently into your meals.

The green juice is extremely healthy; therefore, you may want to continue to drink it daily. In this way, the Sirtfood diet can become a lifestyle change rather than simply the usual one time diet.

Days	Breakfast	Lunch	Dinner
1	Matcha Green Juice	Turmeric Baked Salmon	Baby Spinach Snack
2	Celery Juice	Lamb, Butternut Squash and Date Tagine	Sesame Dip
3	Kale & Orange Juice	Prawn Arrabiata	Rosemary Squash Dip
4	Apple & Cucumber Juice	Sticky Chicken Watermelon Noodle Salad	Bang Chicken Noodle Stir-fry
5	Blueberry Muffins	Baked Potatoes with Spicy Chickpea Stew	Pesto Salmon Pasta Noodles
6	Chocolate Waffles	Fruity Curry Chicken Salad	Bean Spread
7	Lemony Green Juice	Char-grilled Steak	Asian Slaw
8	Buckwheat Porridge	Zuppa Toscana	Sri Lankan-Style Sweet Potato Curry
9	Moroccan Spiced Eggs	Turmeric Chicken & Kale Salad with Honey-Lime Dressing	Salsa Bean Dip
10	Twice Baked Breakfast Potatoes	Kale and Red Onion Dhal with Buckwheat	Orange Carrots
11	Sirt Muesli	Farinata with Zucchini and Shallot	Salmon Burgers

12	Chilaquiles with Gochujang	Kale and Red Onion Dhal with Buckwheat	Mung Beans Snack Salad
13	Spiced Scramble	Zucchini Dumplings	Shrimp with Veggies
14	Chilled Strawberry and Walnut Porridge	Stuffed with Vegetables	Tofu & Veggies Curry
15	Poached Eggs & Rocket (Arugula)	Sponge Beans with Onion	Jackfruit Tortilla Bowl
16	Cheesy Baked Eggs	Beans on the Bird	Parsley Lamb Chops with Kale
17	Strawberry & Nut Granola	Diced Tofu and Lentils	Chickpeas with Swiss chard
18	Strawberry Buckwheat Pancakes	Zucchini Croquettes	Banana Dessert
19	Chocolate Berry Blend	Diced Seitan and Lentils	Grilled Salmon Fillet with Chilies and Avocado Puree
20	Mushroom & Red Onion Buckwheat Pancakes	Tofu Sticks	Beef & Kale Salad
21	Cream of Broccoli & Kale Soup	Crepes Leeks and Mushrooms	Salmon and Capers
22	French Onion Soup	Pizzaiola Steak	Egg Fried Buckwheat
23	Cheesy Buckwheat Cakes	Chicken and Kale with Spicy Salsa	Sautéed Red Cabbage
24	Lentil Soup	Kale and Shiitake Stew	Strawberry Popsicles

			with Chocolate Dip
25	Apple Pancakes	Chili Con Carne	Quinoa Nut and Radicchio Meatballs
26	Matcha Pancakes	Mussels in Red Wine Sauce	Hazelnut Balls
27	Chocolate Muffins	Roast Balsamic Vegetables	Spiced Burger
28	Kale & Mushroom Frittata	Honey Chili Squash	Sweet Potato Hash Brown
29	Kale, Apple, & Cranberry Salad	Baked Cauliflower	Buckwheat Burger
30	Arugula, Strawberry, & Orange Salad	Herb Crepes	Tofu and Buckwheat Salad

Smoothies

117.Lime and Ginger Green Smoothie

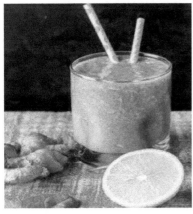

Preparation time: 5 minutes

Cooking time: 5 minutes

Servings: 1

Ingredients:

½ cup dairy free milk

½ cup water

½ teaspoon fresh ginger

½ cup mango chunks

Juice from 1 lime

1 tablespoon dried shredded coconut

1 tablespoon flaxseeds

1 cup spinach

Directions:

Blend together all the ingredients until smooth.

Serve and enjoy!

Nutrition:

Calories 178

Fat 1g

Carbohydrates 7g

Protein 4g

Day 117. Turmeric Strawberry Green Smoothie

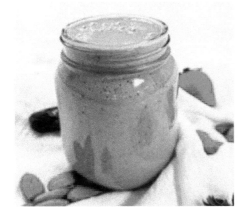

Preparation time: 5 minutes

Cooking time: 5 minutes

Servings: 1

Ingredients:

1 cup kale, stalks removed

1 teaspoon turmeric

1 cup strawberries

½ cup coconut yogurt

6 walnut halves

1 tablespoon raw cacao powder

1-2 mm slice of bird's eye chili

1 cup unsweetened almond milk

1 pitted Medjool date

Directions:

Blend together all the ingredients and enjoy immediately!

Be careful how much almond milk you add so you can choose your favorite consistency.

Nutrition:

Calories 180

Fat 2.2g

Carbohydrates 12g

Protein 4g

Day 118. Sirtfood Wonder Smoothie

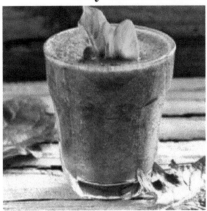

Preparation time: 5 minutes

Cooking time: 10 minutes

Servings: 1

Ingredients:

1 cup arugula (rocket)

2 cups organic strawberries or blueberries

1 cup kale

½ teaspoon matcha green tea

Juice of ½ lemon or lime

3 sprigs of parsley

½ cup of watercress

¾ cup of water

Directions:

Add all the ingredients except matcha to a blender and whizz up until very smooth.

Add the matcha green tea powder and give it a final blitz until well mixed.

Nutrition:

Calories 145

Fat 2g

Carbohydrates 7g

Protein 3g

Day 119. Strawberry Spinach Smoothie

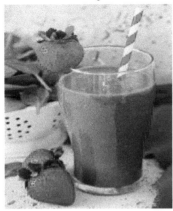

Preparation time: 5 minutes

Cooking time: 5 minutes

Servings: 1

Ingredients:

1 cup whole frozen strawberries

3 cups packed spinach

¼ cup frozen pineapple chunks

1 medium ripe banana, cut into chunks and frozen

1 cup unsweetened milk

1 tablespoon chia seeds

Directions:

Place all the ingredients in a high-powered blender.

Blend until smooth.

Enjoy!

Nutrition:

Calories 266

Fat 8g

Carbohydrates 48g

Protein 9g

Day 120. Berry Turmeric Smoothie

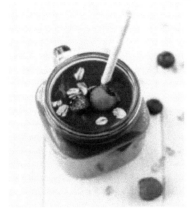

Preparation time: 5 minutes

Cooking time: 5 minutes

Servings: 1

Ingredients:

1 ½ cups frozen mixed berries (blueberries, blackberries and raspberries)

½ teaspoon ground turmeric

2 cups baby spinach

¾ cup unsweetened vanilla almond milk, or milk of choice

½ cup non-fat plain Greek yogurt, or yoghurt of choice

¼ teaspoon ground ginger

2-3 teaspoons honey

3 tablespoons old-fashioned rolled oats

Directions:

Place all the ingredients in a high-powered blender.

Blend until smooth.

Taste and adjust sweetness as desired.

Enjoy immediately!

Nutrition:

Calories 151

Fat 2g

Carbohydrates 27g

Protein 8g

Day 121. Mango Green Smoothie

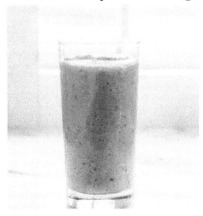

Preparation time: 3 minutes

Cooking time: 5 minutes

Servings: 1

Ingredients:

1 ½ cups frozen mango pieces

1 cup packed baby spinach leaves

1 ripe banana

¾ cup unsweetened vanilla almond milk

Directions:

Place all the ingredients in a blender.

Blend until smooth.

Enjoy!

Nutrition:

Calories 229

Fat 2g

Carbohydrates 72g

Protein 2g

Day 122. Apple Avocado Smoothie

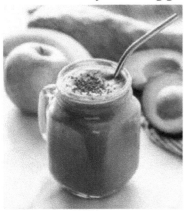

Preparation time: 5 minutes

Cooking time: 5 minutes

Servings: 1

Ingredients:

2 cups packed spinach

½ medium avocados

1 medium apple, peeled and quartered

½ medium bananas, cut into chunks and frozen

½ cup unsweetened almond milk

1 teaspoon honey

¼ teaspoon ground ginger

Small handful of ice cubes

Directions:

In the ordered list, add the almond milk, spinach, avocado, banana, apples, honey, ginger, and ice to a high-powered blender.

Blend until smooth.

Taste and adjust sweetness and spices as desired.

Enjoy immediately!

Nutrition:

Calories 206

Fat 11g

Carbohydrates 15g

Protein 5g

Day 123. Kale Pineapple Smoothie

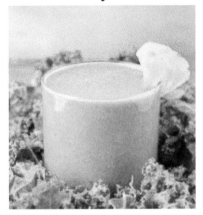

Preparation time: 5 minutes

Cooking time: 5 minutes

Servings: 1

Ingredients:

2 cups lightly packed chopped kale leaves, stems removed

¼ cup frozen pineapple pieces

1 frozen medium banana, cut into chunks

¼ cup non-fat Greek yogurt

2 teaspoons honey

¾ cup unsweetened vanilla almond milk, or any milk of choice

2 tablespoons peanut butter, creamy or crunchy

Directions:

Place all the ingredients in a blender.

Blend until smooth.

Add more milk as needed to reach desired consistency.

Enjoy immediately!

Nutrition:

Calories 187

Fat 9g

Carbohydrates 27g

Protein 8g

Day 124. Blueberry Banana Avocado Smoothie

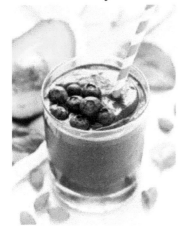

Preparation time: 10 minutes

Cooking time: 10 minutes

Servings: 1

Ingredients:

1 medium ripe banana, peeled

2 cups frozen blueberries

1 cup fresh spinach

1 tablespoon ground flaxseed meal

½ ripe avocados

1 tablespoon almond butter

¼ teaspoon cinnamon

½ cup unsweetened vanilla almond milk

Directions:

Place all the ingredients in your blender in the ordered list: vanilla almond milk, spinach, banana, avocado, blueberries, flaxseed meal, and almond butter.

Blend until smooth.

If you like a thicker smoothie, add a small handful of ice.

Enjoy immediately!

Nutrition:

Calories 298

Fat 14.4g

Carbohydrates 38.1g

Protein 8g

Day 125. Carrot Smoothie

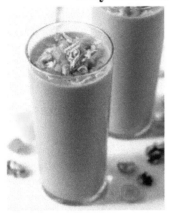

Preparation time: 10 minutes

Cooking time: 10 minutes

Servings: 1

Ingredients:

1 cup chopped carrots

¼ cup frozen diced pineapple

½ cup frozen sliced banana

¼ teaspoon cinnamon

1 tablespoon flaked coconut

½ cup Greek yogurt

2 tablespoons toasted walnuts

Pinch nutmeg

½ cup unsweetened vanilla almond milk, or milk of choice

For topping:

Shredded carrots, coconut, crushed walnuts

Directions:

Add all the ingredients into a blender.

Blend until smooth.

Enjoy immediately, topped with additional shredded carrots, coconut, and crushed walnuts as desired!

Nutrition:

Calories 279

Fat 6g

Carbohydrates 48g

Protein 7g

Day 126. Matcha Berry Smoothie

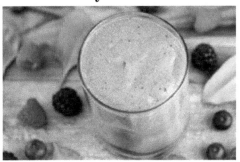

Preparation time: 5 minutes

Cooking time: 5 minutes

Servings: 1

Ingredients:

½ bananas

½-tablespoon matcha powder

1 cup almond milk

1 cup frozen blueberries

¼ teaspoon ground ginger

½ tablespoon chia seeds

¼ teaspoon ground cinnamon

Directions:

In a blender, blend the almond milk, banana, blueberries, matcha powder, chia seeds, cinnamon, and ginger until smooth.

Enjoy immediately!

Nutrition:

Calories 212

Fat 5g

Carbohydrates 34g

Protein 8g

Day 127. Simple Grape Smoothie

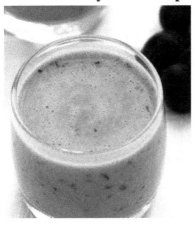

Preparation time: 5 minutes

Cooking time: 5 minutes

Servings: 1

Ingredients:

2 cups red seedless grapes

¼ cup grape juice

½ cup plain yogurt

1 cup ice

Directions:

Add grape juice to the blender. Then add yogurt and grapes. Add the ice last.

Blend until smooth and enjoy!

Nutrition:

Calories 161

Fat 4g

Carbohydrates 39g

Protein 2g

Day 128. Ginger Plum Smoothie

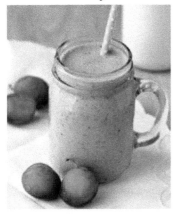

Preparation time: 5 minutes

Cooking time: 5 minutes

Servings: 1

Ingredients:

1 ripe plum, fresh or frozen, pitted but not peeled

½ cup plain yogurt

½ cup orange juice, or other fruit juice

1 teaspoon grated fresh ginger

Directions:

Put all the ingredients in a blender and blend until smooth.

Serve immediately and enjoy!

Nutrition:

Calories 124

Fat 2g

Carbohydrates 26g

Protein 3g

Day 129. Kumquat Mango Smoothie

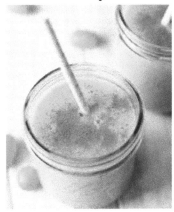

Preparation time: 10 minutes

Cooking time: 5 minutes

Servings: 1

Ingredients:

15 small kumquats

½ mango, peeled and chopped

¾ cup unsweetened almond milk

¼ teaspoon vanilla

½ cup plain yogurt

¼ teaspoon nutmeg

1 tablespoon honey

½ teaspoon ground cinnamon

5 ice cubes

Directions:

Cut the kumquats in half and remove any seeds.

Add all the ingredients to a blender and blend until smooth.

Garnish with another sprinkling of cinnamon, if desired.

Enjoy immediately!

Nutrition:

Calories 116

Fat 2g

Carbohydrates 22g

Protein 5g

Day 130. Cranberry Smoothie

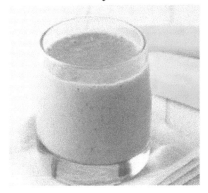

Preparation time: 5 minutes

Cooking time: 5 minutes

Servings: 1

Ingredients:

½ cup frozen cranberries

½ bananas

¼ cup orange juice

¼ cup frozen blueberries

¼ cup low fat Greek yogurt

Directions:

Add all the ingredients to a blender and blend until smooth.

Add a little more orange juice if you prefer it a little thinner. Enjoy immediately!

Nutrition:

Calories 165

Fat 1g

Carbohydrates 31g

Protein 8g

Day 131. Summer Berry Smoothie

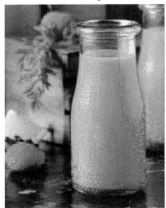

Preparation time: 10 minutes

Cooking time: 10 minutes

Servings: 1

Ingredients:

50g (2oz) blueberries

50g (2oz) strawberries

25g (1oz) blackcurrants

25g (1oz) red grapes

1 carrot, peeled

1 orange, peeled

Juice of 1 lime

Directions:

Place all of the ingredients into a blender and cover them with water. Blitz until smooth.

You can also add some crushed ice and a mint leaf to garnish.

Nutrition:

Calories: 110

Fat: 1 g

Carbohydrates: 20 g

Protein: 2 g

Day 132. Mango, Celery and Ginger Smoothie

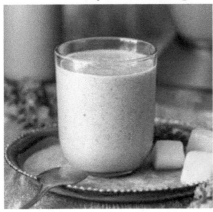

Preparation time: 10 minutes

Cooking time: 10 minutes

Servings: 1

Ingredients:

1 stalk of celery

50g (2oz) kale

1 apple, cored

50g (2oz) mango, peeled, de-stoned and chopped

2.5cm (1 inch) chunk of fresh ginger root, peeled and chopped

Directions:

Put all the ingredients into a blender with some water and blitz until smooth. Add ice to make your smoothie really refreshing.

Nutrition:

Calories: 92

Fat: 3 g

Carbohydrates: 22 g

Protein: 1 g

Day 133. Orange, Carrot and Kale Smoothie

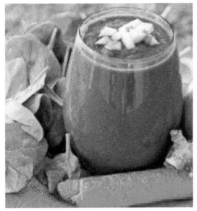

Preparation time: 5 minutes

Cooking time: 5 minutes

Servings: 1

Ingredients:

1 carrot, peeled

1 orange, peeled

1 stick of celery

1 apple, cored

50g (2oz) kale

½ teaspoon matcha powder

Directions:

Place all of the ingredients into a blender and add in enough water to cover them. Process until smooth, serve and enjoy.

Nutrition:

Calories: 150

Fat: 1 g

Carbohydrates: 36 g

Protein: 4 g

Creamy Strawberry and Cherry Smoothie

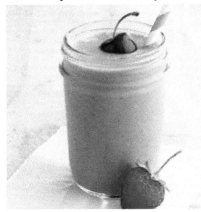

Preparation time: 5 minutes

Cooking time: 5 minutes

Servings: 1

Ingredients:

100g (3½ oz) strawberries

75g (3oz) frozen pitted cherries

1 tablespoon plain full-fat yogurt

175mls (6fl oz) unsweetened soya milk

Directions:

Place all of the ingredients into a blender and process until smooth. Serve and enjoy.

Nutrition:

Calories: 135

Fat: 1 g

Carbohydrates: 25 g

Protein: 3 g

Pineapple and Cucumber Smoothie

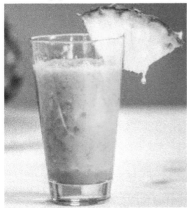

Preparation time: 5 minutes

Cooking time: 5 minutes

Servings: 1

Ingredients:

50g (2oz) cucumber

1 stalk of celery

2 slices of fresh pineapple

2 sprigs of parsley

½ teaspoon matcha powder

Squeeze of lemon juice

Directions:

Place all of the ingredients into blender with enough water to cover them and blitz until smooth.

Nutrition:

Calories: 125

Fat: 1 g

Carbohydrates: 22 g

Protein: 2 g

Day 134. Avocado, Celery and Pineapple Smoothie

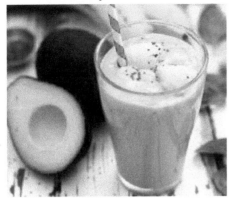

Preparation time: 5 minutes

Cooking time: 5 minutes

Servings: 1

Ingredients:

50g (2oz) fresh pineapple, peeled and chopped

3 stalks of celery

1 avocado, peeled & de-stoned

1 teaspoon fresh parsley

½ teaspoon matcha powder

Juice of ½ lemons

Directions:

Place all of the ingredients into a blender and add enough water to cover them - process until creamy and smooth.

Nutrition:

Calories: 138

Fat: 2 g

Carbohydrates: 25 g

Protein: 5g

Day 135. Mango and Rocket (Arugula) Smoothie

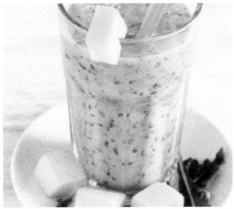

Preparation time: 5 minutes

Cooking time: 5 minutes

Servings: 1

Ingredients:

25g (1oz) fresh rocket (arugula)

150g (5oz) fresh mango, peeled, de-stoned and chopped

1 avocado, de-stoned and peeled

½ teaspoon matcha powder

Juice of 1 lime

Directions:

Place all of the ingredients into a blender with enough water to cover them and process until smooth. Add a few ice cubes and enjoy.

Nutrition:

Calories: 145

Fat: 2 g

Carbohydrates: 21 g

Protein: 5 g

Day 136. Strawberry and Citrus Blend

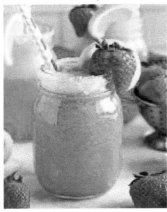

Preparation time: 5 minutes

Cooking time: 5 minutes

Servings: 1

Ingredients:

75g (3oz) strawberries

1 apple, cored

1 orange, peeled

½ avocado, peeled and de-stoned

½ teaspoon matcha powder

Juice of 1 lime

Directions:

Place all of the ingredients into a blender with enough water to cover them and process until smooth. Add ice to make it really refreshing.

Nutrition:

Calories: 112

Fat: 2 g

Carbohydrates: 23 g

Protein: 1 g

Day 137. Orange and Celery Crush

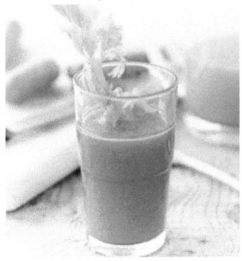

Preparation time: 5 minutes

Cooking time: 5 minutes

Servings: 1

Ingredients:

1 carrot, peeled

3 stalks of celery

1 orange, peeled

½ teaspoon matcha powder

Juice of 1 lime

Directions:

Place all of the ingredients into a blender with enough water to cover them and blitz until smooth. Add crushed ice to make your smoothie really refreshing.

Nutrition:

Calories: 180

Fat: 2 g

Carbohydrates: 25 g

Protein: 3 g

Day 138. Chocolate, Strawberry and Coconut Crush

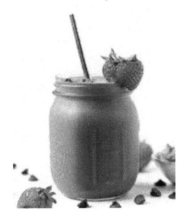

Preparation time: 5 minutes

Cooking time: 5 minutes

Servings: 1

Ingredients:

100mls (3½fl oz) coconut milk

100g (3½oz) strawberries

1 banana

1 tablespoon 100% cocoa powder or cacao nibs

1 teaspoon matcha powder

Directions:

Toss all of the ingredients into a blender and process them to a creamy consistency.

Add a little extra water if you need to thin it a little. Add crushed ice to make your smoothie really refreshing.

Nutrition:

Calories: 220

Fat: 3 g

Carbohydrates: 30 g

Protein: 5 g

Day 139. Banana and Kale Smoothie

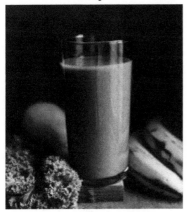

Preparation time: 5 minutes

Cooking time: 5 minutes

Servings: 1

Ingredients:

50g (2oz) kale

1 banana

200mls (7fl oz) unsweetened soya milk

Directions:

Place all of the ingredients into a blender with enough water to cover them and process until smooth. Add ice to make it really refreshing.

Nutrition:

Calories: 189

Fat: 2 g

Carbohydrates: 25 g

Protein: 3 g

Day 140. Cranberry and Kale Crush

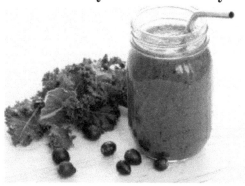

Preparation time: 5 minutes

Cooking time: 5 minutes

Servings: 1

Ingredients:

75g (3oz) strawberries

50g (2oz) kale

120mls (4fl oz) unsweetened cranberry juice

1 teaspoon chia seeds

½ teaspoon matcha powder

Directions:

Place all of the ingredients into a blender and process until smooth. Add some crushed ice and a mint leaf or two for a really refreshing drink.

Nutrition:

Calories: 213

Fat: 1 g

Carbohydrates: 28 g

Protein: 3 g

Day 141. Grape, Celery and Parsley Reviver

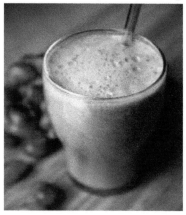

Preparation time: 5 minutes

Cooking time: 5 minutes

Servings: 1

Ingredients:

75g (3oz) red grapes

3 sticks of celery

1 avocado, de-stoned and peeled

1 tablespoon fresh parsley

½ teaspoon matcha powder

Directions:

Place all of the ingredients into a blender with enough water to cover them and blitz until smooth and creamy. Add crushed ice to make it even more refreshing.

Nutrition:

Calories: 253

Fat: 2 g

Carbohydrates: 35 g

Protein: 3 g

Day 142. Grapefruit and Celery Blast

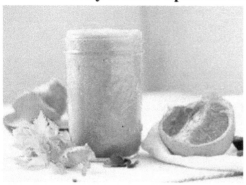

Preparation time: 5 minutes

Cooking time: 5 minutes

Servings: 1

Ingredients:

1 grapefruit, peeled

2 stalks of celery

50g (2oz) kale

½ teaspoon matcha powder

Directions:

Place all the ingredients into a blender with enough water to cover them and blitz until smooth.

Add crushed ice to make it even more refreshing.

Nutrition:

Calories: 220

Fat: 1 g

Carbohydrates: 31 g

Protein: 2 g

Day 143. Tropical Chocolate Delight

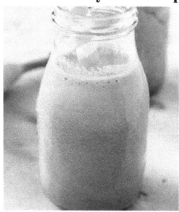

Preparation time: 5 minutes

Cooking time: 5 minutes

Servings: 1

Ingredients:

1 mango, peeled & de-stoned

75g (3oz) fresh pineapple, chopped

50g (2oz) kale

25g (1oz) rocket

1 tablespoon 100% cocoa powder or cacao nibs

150mls (5fl oz) coconut milk

Directions:

Place all of the ingredients into a blender and blitz until smooth. You can add a little water if it seems too thick.

Add crushed ice to make it even more refreshing.

Nutrition:

Calories: 289

Fat: 4 g

Carbohydrates: 37 g

Protein: 3 g

Importance of Sirtfood Diet

We all know dieting can be challenging, especially if you are not used to eating healthy or if you have poor eating habits. Yet it certainly must not be an impossible feat. One of the most significant errors so everyone makes is that they come at the wrong perspective at dieting. It should not be perceived as something that you are using for a "fast remedy" to a weight issue or safety condition. A diet would be a complete lifestyle change that, in a way, would be a thorough redesign of your eating habits. Your food is meant to become your way of life, a method of eating that you hold to for the long haul regularly.

The first idea of having yourself on a diet is choosing to change your eating habits for the better. You'll need to give yourself a long-term dieting target. The easiest way to get you started on your path towards reaching your goal is to continue with tiny, practical improvements.

Now that you've settled on your long-term objective of dieting, the next move is to chart how you can do it. You want this plan to be mapped out one step at a time. It's undoubtedly clear you can tell more about yourself than anyone else, so you can make up your mind to start with either one meal or a whole day. Your enthusiasm will most likely be the determining factor in your diet. It would be best if you remained focused, determined, and motivated until the end. Having support from family, employers, and experts will help keep you focused, but eventually changing your lifestyle is up to you. One great benefit is that all the items you will consume on the program are healthy for you, ensuring the average consumption of vitamins, minerals, and nutrients.

There is still little reason to say that weight reduction is a more successful approach than any other diet regulated by calories. And although the first seven days tend to be tough, the longer-term plan fits everyone. You can continue the fat burning while enjoying your regular favorites by focusing on introducing Sirtfood rich ingredients into your daily meals. Although the Sirtfood diet's first step is very small in calories and nutritionally incomplete, there are no particular safety issues for the normal, stable person given the limited length of the diet.

Yet for someone with diabetes, reducing calories and only consuming juice during the first few days of the diet may cause harmful changes in blood sugar levels. However, even a healthy individual can encounter specific side effects, primarily hunger. Eating only 1,000–1,500 calories a day can leave just about anybody feeling thin, particularly if most of what you're consuming is the juice that's low in fiber, a nutrient that lets you remain complete.

There's no denying that sirtfoods are beneficial for you. They are frequently high in supplements and brimming with sound plant mixes. Besides, examines have related a large number of the foods suggested on the Sirtfood diet with medical advantages. For instance, eating reasonable measures of dim chocolate with a high cocoa substance may bring down the danger of coronary illness and help battle irritation. Drinking green tea may lessen the threat of stroke and diabetes and assist lower with blooding pressure.

Proof of the medical advantages of expanding sirtuin protein levels is fundamental. During fasting or calorie limitation, sirtuin proteins advise the body to consume increasingly fat for vitality and improve insulin. Some proof recommends that sirtuins may likewise assume a job in lessening aggravation, restraining the advancement of tumors, and easing back the improvement of coronary illness and Alzheimer's.

In this way, enhancing sirtuin protein levels in the body will lead to a longer lifespan, or lower risk of disease in humans is obscure. Research is now in progress to create mixes powerful at expanding sirtuin levels in the body. Along these lines, human investigations can start to inspect the impacts of sirtuins on social wellbeing. Up to that point, it's impractical to decide the effects of expanded sirtuin levels. Sirtfoods are usually solid foods.

Eating only a bunch of excellent foods can't meet the entirety of your body's wholesome needs. The Sirtfood diet is superfluously prohibitive and offers no unmistakable, one of a kind medical advantage over some other sort of diet.

The eating routine additionally requires drinking up to three green juices for each day. Although juices can be a decent wellspring of nutrients and minerals, they are additionally a wellspring of sugar and contain practically none of the sound fiber that whole foods grew from the ground do. Tasting on juice all through the entire day is an ill-conceived notion for both your glucose and your teeth.

Also, because the eating regimen is restricted in calories and food decisions, it is more than likely insufficient in protein, nutrients, and minerals, particularly during the primary stage.

Even though the first period of the Sirtfood diet is low in calories and healthfully inadequate, there are no genuine security worries for the healthy, solid grown-up thinking about the eating regimen's brief term. For somebody with diabetes, calorie limitation, and drinking, for the most part, squeeze for the initial not many days of the eating routine may cause risky changes in glucose levels. Even a stable individual may encounter some reactions, mostly hunger. Because of the low-calorie levels and prohibitive food decisions, this eating regimen might be hard to adhere to for the whole three weeks. It gets unfeasible and impractical for some individuals, but it might be a good idea to add Sirtfood to your regular diet over time.

Combining the Sirtfood Diet with Exercise for Ultimate Success

Often, when trying to lose weight, people will attempt to increase exercise while eating less. However, this plan alone is often ineffective. People will often work hard week after week without seeing the results. The good news is that the Sirt diet is excellent for increasing weight loss with exercise, as the Sirtfoods and caloric restriction can mimic the fat loss properties of fasting. This allows you to lose weight without burdening yourself with excessive exercise.

When we are trying to lose weight and excessively increase the amount of exercise we do, the truth is that it backfires. Sure, exercise in moderation has many health benefits. But, just like everything, exercise can be done in excess. When this is done, it can reduce the amount of weight you can lose. How is this possible? It is because people will frequently overeat to make up for the calories lost through exercise. But, when this happens, you are undoing the beneficial effects of dieting, because you are now eating more than you should for your body type.

Along with increasing hunger and food consumption, excessive exercise even alters your hormonal balance. This can cause weight loss disaster, as hormones are a precarious balance, and when they become out of balance, it messes with the entire body. While hormones can increase your weight loss, when you over-exercise yourself, the hormones go in the opposite way of what you want, preventing you from losing weight.

By exercising on the Sirtfood diet, you can experience similar weight loss results to those experienced when exercising while intermittent fasting. By looking at scientific studies on intermittent fasting and exercise, we can get a better picture of what is going on in the body and the specific results of your hard work. These studies show that you can lose more weight than you usually would from exercise and dieting, but you can do so without excessive exercise that would push your body past its limits. This will allow your hormones to stay in a healthy balance, prevent overeating, and overall improve your daily life.

Of course, while exercise is much effective when you are on the Sirt diet, it is always important to listen to your body and its individual needs. This is because every person's body has its limits, and if you don't listen to the signals, you can go past your limits and wind up with an injury or practicing exercise in excess.

Not all forms of exercise affect the body in the same way. Some types of exercise are short bursts of high-intensity exercise. The good news is that there are other exercises perfect for the Sirt diet, namely, cardio. Unlike the previously mentioned exercises, cardio isn't an all-out intense and fast-paced exercise. Instead, cardio allows you to pace yourself, as long as you get your heart rate up. This is good for increasing your general strength and stamina, along with improving your heart health. Many experts recommend fasting for at least a few hours before practicing a cardio workout, as eating beforehand will interfere with proper digestion and lessen nutrient absorption.

There are many types of cardio to do, to improve your strength, endurance, protect your heart health, and lose more weight. These are great options, even when you are in the first phase of the Sirt diet. Keep in mind that whenever you are exercising, you should listen to your body and its individual needs. This is especially true when you are dieting and might have less stamina than usual. Depending on how much energy you have, you might practice one of these cardio exercises for just a minute or two. But, if you have more energy, you can create an entire workout using various methods listed here.

Jog in Place

By staying in a stationary position while you jog, you can exercise in a space-limited environment. While the space you are in may be small, the exercise itself is an easy and accessible way to warm up your muscles and get your heart pumping. Even if you plan on doing more intense exercises, by starting with jogging in place, you can reduce the likelihood of injury, as any physical trainer will tell you warm-ups are essential.

While jogging in place is a great way to warm up for more intense exercises, you still shouldn't jump right into the exercise. Doing this can increase the risk of energy. Instead, start by marching in place. As your muscles begin to warm up, you can slowly alternate into a jog.

Jumping Jacks

Many people have used jumping jacks as a simple and straight-forward form of cardio since childhood. With this method, all you have to do is jump wide and spread out your arms above your head, then jump again to bring your legs and arms back together. This is great, as it works out the muscles in your body, such as your legs, core, and arms. Without having any special equipment, space requirements, or skills, you can usually burn about one-hundred calories in just ten minutes with jumping jacks.

Although it is important to remember that like all exercises, jumping jacks won't work for everyone. More specifically, they are high-impact, meaning they can cause joint pain for individuals with joint illnesses or injuries.

Jump Rope

With just a little rope, you can create a great rhythmic exercise of jump rope, which can even be fun. Many children practice this, not for exercise, but to pass the time. If you want to enjoy it more, try singing songs or creating rhymes as you jump. Keep in mind that you should practice this in a larger room or outdoors, to avoid breaking any fragile objects in the home.

Burpees

If you are up for a challenge, then burpees are for you. With this form of exercise, you squat low to the floor before jumping your body into a plank position. You then jump back to a squat before standing up. For a series of burpees, you do multiple times, often at a rapid pace. While this type of exercise is more difficult and can cause more impact to the joints, if your body can do it, it is a great way to give yourself a full-body workout.

Squat Jumps

If you have strong joints, specifically knees then, squat jumps are a great way to burn a lot of calories quickly, strengthen your legs, and increase your heart rate. While these do require a lot of energy and strong joints, they don't require any especially strong skills. This means that even for beginners, they are relatively simple. If you want to try burpees, but they are a little too difficult for you, try practicing first with the squat jump. As you better excel at the squat jump, you will find burpees slightly less difficult.

Mountain Climbers

To practice mountain climbers, imagine you are climbing an incline. When you do this, your knees come close to your hands as your feet look for a foothold. You can work out your body in a similar way, without the actual incline. To do this, you first get into a push-up position.

From there, you run your knees in and out, toward and away from your hands. To prevent from causing injury, start slow as your muscles warm-up and gradually increase the speed.

Bear Crawl Push-Ups

While this type of push-up is relatively simple, it is harder than it looks! You begin by squatting on the floor. You then walk your hands out away from you on the floor until you are in the push-up position. Once you get in this position, you walk your hands back again, which allows you to slowly stand back up, much like you would see a bear doing.

This is a great high-intensity cardio exercise that helps get your heart rate up, improving your strength and endurance with practice. You will quickly find that just a for repetitions of this can have quite an effect.

Kickboxing

A great way to get your heart rate up, increase strength and endurance, get out any anger or aggression and practice self-defense is kickboxing. While it is most effective if you have a bag to practice against, you can even practice against the air. If you are getting into kickboxing, you can try practicing against the air or using a bag at the gym, and as you develop more skill, you may even decide to purchase your bag for at-home use. While this type of exercise does require more knowledge, as you need to learn basic information and punches and kicks, it isn't overly difficult to get started.

Staircase Exercise

Staircase exercises are used for a variety of cardio and strength training exercises. There are countless types and variations that you can use for whatever muscles you want to work out on a given day. The great news is that you don't even need an actual case of stairs, as you can use a fitness platform or even a stepping stool to practice many of these exercises.

While you can always use a variety of creative staircase exercises, if you have a staircase at home or nearby at a park, you can always walk or jog up and down them for an effective workout.

Cardio Play

There are countless ways you can incorporate cardio into your everyday life in a fun and playful ways. This could include riding a bike, using a pair of skates, playing a game of frisbee or soccer, or simply enjoying a walk or job in a relaxing park or around a pond.

By creating your cardio circuit, you can maximize an effective workout with all of your favorite cardio exercises. This allows you to practice them in specific orders and intervals to keep your body moving, increase your stamina, and work out a larger variety of muscles.

Conclusion

Diet research is all about these sirtfoods, a collection of recently identified daily plant foods rich in a chemical compound known as 'sirtuin' activators. These sirtuin activators are a kind of protein that turns into the body's 'skinny gene' pathway. These slender pathways are the same ones that are most often stimulated by fasting and exercise, which help the body lose weight, increase muscle mass, and increase fitness. Sirtfood stimulates the genes of sirtuin, which is reported to influence the body's ability to burn fat and boost the metabolic system.

Like other short-term diets, the sirtfood plan offers recipes and advice on how to keep the weight you lose within the first week while attempting to adopt sirtfood as part of a healthy and balanced lifestyle. Dieters consume two natural drinks a day for the early three days, including spinach, celery, rocket, parsley, lemon, and green tea, and eat one meal.

The emphasis shifts to eating 'normally' again after the initial fasting stage; however, high the consumption of balanced sirt foods may be. The initial step of juicing and fasting is just unusual for someone who might want to turn a few pounds immediately. The general approach of the sirtfoods diet is to incorporate healthy foods into your diet to improve your well-being and strengthen your immune system over time. So, while the first seven days seem to be hardcore, the longer-term plan works for everyone. You will start burning fat when you enjoy your daily treats by focusing on adding rich sirtfood ingredients to your daily meals.

The biggest plus is that this lifestyle actively promotes red wine, dark chocolate, and coffee. The compounds that make up our favorite treats are abundant in sirtuin actuators. Participants never get hungry, which suggests that it's perfect for someone who can't get through a regular cleaning day without feeling like they're going to die because they don't have a vast mac right away. The first week of the plan is very intense.

Sirtfood is almost all healthy choices, and due to its antioxidant or anti-inflammatory properties, it can even produce some health benefits. This diet may be challenging to maintain for three weeks due to low-calorie levels and restrictive food choices. Connect this to the high initial cost of purchasing a juicer, a book, and other odd and expensive items, as well as the time cost of cooking various foods and juices. This lifestyle is unfeasible and impractical for a few.

The sirtfood diet is made of nutritious food, so it's not a proper dietary habit. These hypotheses and safety arguments are, not to mention, based on extensive extrapolations of sparse empiric facts. Although it's not a terrible thing to attach any sirt products to the diet and even provide some health benefits, the diet itself seems to be another fad. Save your money and instead skip to make your lifestyle safe, long-term improvements.

Remember to keep on going and never quit, the best things come to those who are patient and persevere despite the difficulties. You'll find out that this diet is much easier than you think. Do not only focus on results but enjoy the journey. This is the best way to get the most out of this program.

Lightning Source UK Ltd.
Milton Keynes UK
UKHW050842280121
377828UK00002B/60